EXPLORE YOUR THYROID

An essential and summarised guide on thyroid function , anatomy, diseases and dieting.

COPYRIGHT © Moulios Anastasios 2019. All rights reserved.

All rights reserved. No part of this publication may be reproduced, distributed, stored in a retrieval system in any form or by any means, including photocopying, recording, or other electronic or mechanical methods.

INTRODUCTION	4
CHAPTER 1: ANATOMY OF THYROID GLAND	5
CHAPTER 2: FUNCTION OF THYROID GLAND	10
CHAPTER 3: METABOLISM OF THYROID HORMONES	15
CHAPTER 4: BIOLOGICAL ACTIVITY OF THYROID HORMONES	18
CHAPTER 5: CONTROL OF THE ACTIVITIES OF THYROID GLAND	21
CHAPTER 6: THYROID FUNCTIONS AND IMMUNE SYSTEM	30
CHAPTER 7: LABORATORY TESTS FOR DIAGNOSIS OF DISEASES OF THYROID	36
CHAPTER 8: DISORDERS OF THYROID FUNCTION	38
CHAPTER 9: THYROID DIET PLAN	120

Introduction

The thyroid gland is one of the most important glands of the endocrine system and plays an important role in the normal tissue development as well as the subsequent metabolic pathway. It consists of 2 lobes (right and left) connected to the isthmus.

The thyroid gland produces three hormones: 1) thyroxine or tetraiodothyronine (T4) and 2) triiodothyronine (T3) regulating the metabolism of all tissues, and 3) calcitonin that lowers blood calcium levels. Thyroid hormone synthesis and secretion is regulated by thyroid stimulating hormone (TSH) produced in the pituitary gland, which in turn is dependent on secretion of thyroglobulin hormone (TRH) produced in the hypothalamus.

Thyroid gland pathology includes: 1) thyroid growth abnormalities; 2) conditions that cause hyperthyroidism; 3) diseases that cause hypothyroidism; 4) thyroiditis; 5) thyroid cancer.

Thyroid cancer is the most common cancer of endocrine glands and accounts for 1-2% of all tumors. It is usually treated with total or partial thyroidectomy followed by diagnostic scanning by scintigraphy.

Chapter 1: Anatomy of thyroid gland

The thyroid gland is the largest endocrine gland in the body. It is butterfly-shaped. It is located in front of the trachea and extends over the middle of the thyroid cartilage of the larynx. It consists of two lateral lobes, the right and the left lobe connected to a central part, the isthmus. On the back surface of the gland are the parathyroid glands.

The weight of the gland at birth amounts to 2-3 grams. During puberty it reaches 10-15 grams. Its maximum weight is obtained during adulthood, 20 to 30 grams. After his 60th birthday, his weight is gradually decreasing. It is older in women, as well as during pregnancy and lactation. The gland has a deep brownish red color. Its normal volume is 10-30 ml.

Each lobe has a conical shape. Thyroid glandular lobes are 4 to 8 cm long, 2 to 4 cm wide and 1.5 to 2.5 cm thick each and are attached near their base to the isthmus of the thyroid gland. The right lobe is slightly wider than the left. The lobes extend obliquely up and down, adhere to the trachea, the carotid and thyroid cartilage with loose connective tissue and are connected by ligaments from the capsule surrounding the organ. The lobes are triangular in cross-section: their anterior surfaces are convex and their inner surfaces adjacent to the trachea and larynx are respectively concave. Their posterior lips are on both sides in contact with large cervical vessels. The upper poles of the lobes extend to the oblique line of the thyroid cartilage and the lower poles to the trachea. Muscles under the bone partially cover the thyroid gland. The medial or pre-tracheal cervical fascia extends over the thyroid gland and continues beyond it.

The thyroid gland is surrounded by a strong fibrous capsule consisting of two layers. The single layer is the inner connective tissue capsule that is thin and adheres tightly to the parenchyma of the gland, delivering connective tissue membranes with vessels within the gland that divide the gland into smaller and larger lobes. The outer capsule is stronger and is considered part of the pre-cerebral cervical fascia. The space between the two loose bonded layers of the capsule is filled with loose connective tissue and contains large vascular branches and at the back of the parathyroid gland. The posterior and lateral surfaces of the outer capsule are attached to the connective tissue of the angiotensive cervical bundle.

Arteries - Thyroid gland is large, calculated at 4-6 ml / min / gr. The right lobe has a richer blood supply than the left, is usually larger and grows more often nodules. Thyroid vasculature is mainly caused by two pairs of arteries, the upper and lower thyroid artery and sometimes also the middle thyroid artery. The upper thyroid artery is the first branch of the external carotid artery. It curves upwards and delivers the upper laryngeal artery to the upper poles of the lateral lobes. Adjacent the anterior upper and lateral parts of the thyroid gland. The lower thyroid artery, branch of the thyroidal shaft. It covers the lower, rear and inner parts of the organ.

Veins - Thyroid veins form a rich lattice located on the surface of the gland. The veins that drain the thyroid gland expose the upper gland to the upper thyroid vein that expels to the internal jugular vein. The lower thyroid veins are derived from the single thyroid gland, located in the pre-tracheal space and flowing behind the sternum.

Lymph - separated into those that drain the upper and lower glands and pass through the upper and middle fate of the gland to the outside cervical lymph nodes along the inner septum. The lingual lymph nodes are associated with upper lymph nodes.

Nerves - Thyroid neurosis is double as it comes from the sympathetic and parasympathetic system. Adrenergic post-transglinic sympathetic fibers are vasomotor, derived from the upper and sympathetic cervical ganglion and enter the gland together with its arteries. The pre-angiogenic parasympathetic fibers come from the vagus nerve and reach the glands of the laryngeal nerve. They also nerve the blood vessels of the gland, regulate blood circulation and indirectly affect its secretory function.

Each lobe consists of follicles. The follicles are the smallest complete thyroid function. They are spherical or tubular in shape and are formed from an epithelial layer with obstructive connections and distinct cellular boundaries. The height of the epithelium depends on the activity of the thyroid gland. Epithelial cells are flat or cuboid when large amounts of excretion are stored in the gland. Cylindrical is during discharge.

In addition to the follicular cells, the thyroid gland also contains parafollicular cells or C cells. Cells are located in the intercellular connective tissue as well as dispersed between the polarized, follicular epithelial cells, where they are located between the basement membrane but do not reach the lumen of the pocket. These cells produce calcitonin.

Chapter 2: Function of thyroid gland

The primary function of the thyroid is the production of the iodine-containing thyroid hormones, triiodothyronine (T_3) and thyroxine (T_4) and the peptide hormone calcitonin. T_3 is so named because it contains three atoms of iodine per molecule and T_4 contains four atoms of iodine per molecule.

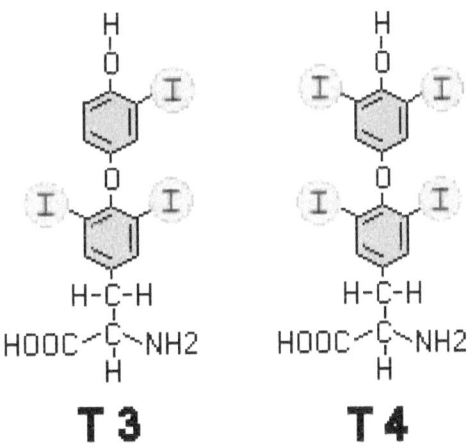

Image 2: Thyroid hormones.

The thyroid hormones have a wide range of effects on the human body. Thyroxine or tetraiodothyronine (T4) and triiodothyronine (T3) promote body growth during endometrial pregnancy, maturation of various tissues and still plays a vital role in all human metabolic functions for the rest of his/her life. In small quantities reverse triiodothyronine (rT3) is produced, which is inactive. Of the parafollicular cells, calcitonin is produced and its function is the decrease the calcium levels in blood.

Thyroxine (T4) and triiodothyronine (T3) are iodinated tyrosine derivatives that are abundant in the gland. Thyroxine consists of two phenolic rings and the alanine molecule as side chain. The two rings are joined at an angle of 110 ° and the outside is in a plane perpendicular to the plane of the inner ring. This structure and the two iodine atoms bearing each ring give thyroxine its specific biological effects.

Synthesis and secretion of thyroid hormones is regulated by:
- the basic raw material that is iodine, which is taken up by thyroid cells from the circulation.
- The integrity of the endothyroid enzyme systems responsible for hormone synthesis and thyroglobulin synthesis.
- thyroid stimulating hormone (TSH) secreted by the anterior pituitary gland and in turn is dependent on the secretion of TRH produced in the hypothalamus.
- The level of thyroid hormones due to the reciprocal action they exert on TSH and the action of tissues that convert T4 to the more active T3.

Iodine: At the heart of thyroid function is iodine, which is the main raw material for the synthesis of thyroid hormones. The uptake is from food or water, in the form of iodine or iodide ion in the form of covalent compounds (iodide), which is converted to iodine in the stomach. Over millennia, iodine from the soil was transferred to the water in the oceans, resulting in mountainous and inland areas have limited stocks, while the element is abundant in coastal areas. The thyroid collects and traps iodine and synthesizes and stores thyroid hormones in thyroglobulin, compensating for the deprivation of iodine.

The average daily dose of iodine intake from food ranges from 120 to 500 μg. Iodine-rich foods include lobster, shrimp and some fish. For adults the mean daily iodine intake is 150 μg, during pregnancy and breastfeeding is 200 μg, in the first year of life is 50 μg, for ages 1-6 is 90 μg and for 6-12 is 120 μg. If iodine uptake is less than 50 μg / day, the gland cannot maintain adequate hormonal secretion resulting in thyroid (goiter) and hypothyroidism. Other sources of iodine in the diet include iodinated salt, vitamin, metal, iodine-containing medicines.

The metabolic cycle of iodine is as follows: Iodine is rapidly absorbed from the gastrointestinal tract and distributed to extracellular fluids as well as to secretions of the salivary glands, breast and stomach. Although the concentration of inorganic iodine in the extracellular fluid reservoir varies depending on iodine uptake, the iodine ion of the extracellular fluid is usually quite low due to its rapid removal through thyroid uptake and renal clearance.

In the thyroid gland, the iodine ion is transported by non-active transfer from the serum through the thyroid membrane base membrane. The thyroid assumes about 115 µg of iodine ion every 24 hours. Approximately 75 µg of iodine ion are used for the synthesis of hormones and stored in thyroglobulin. The rest escapes to the extracellular fluid reservoir. Iodine uptake is done with a thyroid pump. The thyroid reservoir of organic iodine represents a stock of hormones to protect the body during periods of iodine deficiency. From this storage tank, about 75 micrograms of hormonal iodine are released daily in the circulation.

Composition of Thyroid Hormones: Production of thyroid hormones and their release into circulation follows these biosynthetic stages.

a. Synthesis and storage of thyroglobulin.

b. Active transfer of iodine ion inside the thyroid cell (trapping of iodine).

c. Iodine oxidation, iodination of thyroglobulin and formation of iodotyrosines.

d. The coupling of iodotyrosines and the formation of thyroid hormones.

e. Reabsorption of thyroglobulin, thyroid hormone release and apoptosis of iodotyrosines.

Chapter 3: Metabolism of thyroid hormones

After the thyroid hormones enter the blood, they pass through the liver, which is a storage and metabolic laboratory for them. The liver has the ability to selectively retain thyroxine, so that its concentration is three times that of the blood. It is estimated that 30% of the extracellular amount of T4 and 5% of T3 is in the liver, which in this way can feed thyroid hormones periphery faster than thyroid.

In addition to its storage capacity, the liver represents the most important locus of metabolic transformation of thyroid hormones and the source of binding protein production.

Thyroid hormones are metabolized in 3 ways. First, with aphibia that progressively removes all iodine atoms from the T4 molecule and T3.

A second way of metabolism is demineralization that occurs mainly in the kidneys and decarboxylation, leading to the formation of tetraioded and triioded derivatives of pyrophosphate (TETRAC and TRIAC) and lactic acid.

A third way of metabolism is glucuronic acid (especially in the liver) and lactic acid (mainly in the kidneys) and the formation of metabolites that circulate in the blood and are excreted with bile, stools and urine.

The anomalies of thyroid hormones and especially thyroxine, which is the main hormone secretion of the thyroid, is absolutely associated with their activity, and therefore the function of the enzymes that act on it acts as an important regulating factor for thyroid hormone activity.

The point of the thyroxine dyspnoea is also of great importance for the action of thyroid hormones because removal of an iodine molecule from the first ring of T4 generates T3, which is 3-8 times the target, stronger than T4, while dissociation of a molecule from the second ring results in the formation of the inactive reverse T3 (rT3).

There are at least 3 deiodinases that have different tissue localization, different action substrates, and different behavior in drugs and diseases.

A type of deiodinase that is abundant in the liver and kidneys and in smaller amounts in other tissues, converts T4 to T3 and is responsible for the amount of T3 that circulates in the blood and reaches the tissues to act. This deiodinase is increased in hyperthyroidism and is inhibited by propylthiouracil and not by the imidazole derivatives. Its molecule contains selenium and for this reason the selenium of food is related to the activity of the enzyme.

The second type of deiodinase is found in the pituitary and the brain and is believed to regulate the intracellular level of T3 in pituitary and nerve cells. It is sensitive to T4 which inhibits it and thus prevents the excessive production and action of T3 in case of T4 hypersecretion. Propylthiouracil does not act on this deiodinase.

The third deiodinase is in the placenta and CNS and inactivates T4 and T3 by converting the first to reverse T3 (rT3) and the second to the inactive diiodotyrosin.

The biological significance of the type and extent of metabolic transformations undergoing thyroid hormones is obvious. The rate, e.g. Thyroxine converted to more active T3 or inactive rT3 or little active TRIAC and TETRAC is related to the intensity with which its biological activity manifests itself.

Under normal conditions, 34% of T4, all of which comes from the thyroid, is converted to T3 and 42% is metabolized to rT3. Thus, the majority of T3 (80%) and almost all of rT3 (95%) is derived from thyroxine. Certain pathological conditions, such as fasting, hepatic and renal failure and pharmacological factors, affect the above transformation in favor of rT3. Increased amounts of rT3 also have newborns.

Chapter 4: Biological activity of thyroid hormones

The resulting anomalies of the removal of thyroid gland are:
1. Decrease in oxygen consumption
2. Inhibition of body growth
3. Suspension of ripening of certain organisms
4. Poor development of CNS function
5. Disorders of the cardiovascular and gastrointestinal tract, metabolism of albumins, fats and carbohydrates.

The responsibility of thyroid hormones for the onset of these disorders is evidenced by the fact that they are all recruited or redeemable by the timely administration of thyroid hormones.

1. Oxygen consumption by tissues. The most important action of thyroid hormones is to increase the consumption of oxygen by the tissues. This action is all but particularly evident in the heart muscle and gastric mucosa. Exception is the brain, the genital glands and the spleen, which show no change in oxygen consumption under the influence of thyroid hormones. The biological effect does not appear immediately, but after a latency of several hours and increases in intensity over a few days. Triiodothyronine acts more strongly and faster than thyroxine, but the duration of its action is shorter.

2. Action on physical growth. Physical growth, especially bone growth in childhood, is among other factors and under the influence of thyroid hormones. Thyroid deficiency or destruction results in inhibition of growth and timely administration of thyroid hormones restores normal growth.

3. Action in maturation. The final conformation of certain tissues is assisted by thyroid hormones.

4. Action in the development of the central nervous system. The development, differentiation and organization of the central nervous system during fetal life and after birth are influenced by thyroid hormones. Human congenital hypothyroidism entails impaired brain function, which is reversible when timely thyroid hormones are administered.

5. Action in sympathetic system. Thyroid hormones increase the β-adrenergic receptors of the heart, skeletal muscles, adipose tissue and other tissues. In addition, they are believed to enhance the action of catecholamines at a post-doping site. The result is the supraventricularity which is due to most of the manifestations of overproduction of thyroid hormones during hyperthyroidism and which is inhibited by beta-receptor blocking drugs.

6. Action in the cardiovascular system. Thyroid hormones exert a strong chronotropic and inotropic effect on the cardiovascular system. They increase β-receptors and G proteins, stimulate the expression of heavy myosin α chains and enhance muscle contraction and exert other intracellular actions. The result is tachycardia and increased cardiac output during hyperthyroidism.

7. Action in the gastrointestinal system. Thyroid hormones increase bowel motility. This action is manifested in the extreme forms of hyperthyroidism and hypothyroidism with frequent stools and constipation respectively.

8. Action on the metabolism of fats and carbohydrates.

Particularly evident is the action of thyroid hormones in synthesis, liver degradation and cholesterol excretion. The effect of this action is to reduce blood cholesterol.

Thyroid hormones increase the absorption of glucose from the intestine and speed up degradation of insulin. At the same time, they increase the glycogenolytic effect of adrenaline. Because of these effects, hyperthyroidism is associated with an increase in blood sugar, although thyroid hormones also increase the consumption of glucose by the tissues.

Chapter 5: Control of the activities of thyroid gland

Thyroid growth and function and peripheral actions of thyroid hormones are controlled by at least four mechanisms:

• The main mode of adjustment is exercised by the hypothalamic-pituitary-thyroid axis, in which the hypothalamic thyroid stimulating hormone (TRH) stimulates synthesis and release from the anterior pituitary of the thyroid stimulating hormone (TSH), which in turn stimulates the thyroid stimulating hormone increase and hormone secretion of the thyroid gland.

• The action of pituitary deiodinase and peripheral tissue deiodinations.

• Thyroid cells show self-regulation of their function depending on the iodine they employ.

• Thyroid hormones exert a reciprocal negative adjustment.

<u>Thyrothropin releasing hormone</u>

The thyrotropin releasing hormone is a tripeptide, pyroglutamic acid-histidine-prolineamide, which is composed of neurons of hypopathic and supraventricular nuclei. It is stored in the inner lining of the hypothalamus and then transferred from the pituitary portal vein through the stomach to the anterior pituitary, where it controls the synthesis and release of TSH. TRH is also found in other parts of the hypothalamus, brain and spinal cord, where it can function as a neurotransmitter. The pre-proTRH gene in humans is based on chromosome 3 and contains a 3.3 kb transcriptional unit, which encodes six TRH molecules. The gene also encodes other neuropeptides which may be biologically significant. In the anterior pituitary, TRH binds to specific receptors in the thyroid and lactor membrane (PRL secreting cells), stimulating the synthesis and release of TSH and prolactin. Thyroid hormones cause a slow decrease in TRH receptors in the pituitary, reducing the response to TRH. Conversely, estrogens increase TRH receptors, thus increasing the pituitary sensitivity in TRH.

The response of thyroid to TRH occurs in two ways: First, it stimulates the release of stored hormone and secondly it stimulates gene activity, thus increasing hormonal synthesis. The TRH receptor (TRH-R) belongs to the family of receptors that possess seven membrane-bound, GTP-binding and protein-bound receptors. The TRH-R gene is seated on chromosome 8. Large glycoprotein hormones, such as TSH and LH, bind to the extracellular fragments of their receptors, but TRH, which is a small peptide, binds to the TRM-R third trans-membrane strand . After binding to its thyrotropin receptor, TRH activates a G protein, which in turn activates phospholipase c to hydrolyze inositol phosphatidyl 4,5 diphosphate (PIP2) to 1,4,5 inositol triphosphate (IP3). IP3 stimulates the release of intracellular $Ca+$, thus causing the first explosive phase of hormonal secretion. At the same time, 1.2 diaglycerol is produced, which is considered responsible for the second and prolonged phase of hormonal secretion. Increases in intracellular $Ca+$ and protein C may contribute to increased transcriptional activity. TRH also stimulates the glycosylation of TSH, which is essential for complete biological activity of the hormone. Thus patients with hypothalamic tumors and hypothyroidism may have measurable TSH, which is not glycosylated and therefore biologically inactive.

Specific in vitro and in vivo studies have shown that T3 directly inhibits transcription of the pre-preTRH gene and therefore the composition of TRH in the hypothalamus. Since T4 is converted to T3 within peptideterrheic neurons (peptides secrete neurons), it is also an effective inhibitor of TRH synthesis and secretion.

TRH is rapidly metabolised, with a half-life after intravenous administration, about 5 minutes. Plasma TRH levels in healthy subjects are very low and range from 25-100 pg / ml.

TSH secretion, stimulated by TRH, takes place throughout 24 hours. In healthy subjects, the mean thrust height of TSH is about 0.6 μU / ml and the mean frequency is one thrust every 1.8 hours. Therefore, healthy individuals are observed to have a circadian rhythm, with maximum TSH values occurring during the night, usually between midnight and 4am. These peak values are not related to sleep, food intake, or the secretion of other pituitary hormones. Possibly, this rate is controlled by a hypothalamic neural impulse generator, which directs the composition of TRH to hyperactive and supraventricular nuclei. In patients with hypothyroidism, the thrust intensity and night-time rise of the level are much higher than normal, while in patients with hyperthyroidism, both fever and night waves are significantly suppressed.

In experimental animals and in newborn infants, exposure to cold increases the secretion of TRH and TSH, but is not seen in adults.

Certain hormones and drugs can alter the composition and release of TRH. The secretion of TRH is stimulated by low T4 and T3 serum values, alpha adrenergic agonists and arginine vasopressin. In contrast, TRH secretion is inhibited by the increase in T3 and T4 and by alpha adrenergic blockade.

Intravenous administration of TRH to humans, at a loading dose of 200-500 µg, causes a rapid increase in serum TSH every 3-5 times, reaching the maximum after 30 minutes and a total duration of 2-3 hours. In patients with primary hypothyroidism in whom the basal TSH value is high - a high response is observed. The response is suppressed in patients with hyperthyroidism, in those with autologous autonomic goiter nodules, in patients treated with high doses of thyroxine and in patients with pituitary hypothyroidism. In a patient with hypothalamic lesion, TSH's partial response to TRH is a complete pituitary. TRH is also found in islet cells of the pancreas, gastrointestinal tract, placenta, heart and prostate, testicles and ovaries. In these peripheral tissues, TRH mRNA is not inhibited by T3.

Thyrothropin: Thyroid hormone, or thyreotropin (TSH) is a glycoprotein synthesized and secreted by thyroid cells of the anterior pituitary gland. It has a molecular weight of about 28 kDa and consists of 2 non-covalently linked subunits, α and β. The α subunit is for the other two glycoproteins of the pituitary, FSH and LH, as well as for the placental hormone hCG. The β subunit is different for each glycoprotein hormone and ensures the specificity of binding and biological activity. The human α subunit has a 92 amino acid and contains 2 oligosaccharide chains. The β subunit of TSH has a 112 amino acid and contains a oligosaccharide chain. Glycosylation takes place in the giant endoplasmic reticulum and the Golgi system of thyrotrophic cells, where glucose, manizzine, fucose, and finally divine or sialic acid residues are bound to the core. The function of these carbohydrate residues is not clear, but it is thought likely to increase the biological activity of TSH and alter the rate of metabolic clearance. For example, de-glycosylated TSH binds to its receptor, but its biological activity is significantly reduced and the rate of metabolic clearance is significantly increased.

    The human α subunit gene is based on chromosome 6 and the β subunit gene on chromosome 1. Several families with a point mutation in the TSH β subunit gene have been reported, resulting in the production of a β subunit that is not bound with α subunit to produce the biologically active TSH. The disorders were autonomic and the clinical picture was that of hypothyroidism.

TSH is the major factor in controlling thyroid growth and synthesis and secretion of thyroid hormones. This is achieved by binding to a specific receptor for TSH (TSH-R) in the thyroid cell membrane and the cAMP adenylyl cyclase system G and the phospholipase C system. The TSH receptor gene in humans is based on chromosome 14q3. TSH-R is a single-chain glycoprotein, containing 764 amino acids. Like the TRH receptor in the anterior pituitary, TSH-R in the thyroid follicular cell belongs to the family of receptors that cross the membrane 7 times, GTP-coupled and protein-bound. Structurally, it can be divided into two subunits: subunit A, which contains 397 amino acids and represents the extracellular ligand binding domain and subunit B, which comprises the intra membrane and intracellular portion of the receptor and participates in the stimulation of thyroid cell growth, the synthesis of thyroid hormones and their extraction. TSH-R is unique because it has binding sites not only for TSH but for TSH-receptor-stimulating antibodies [TSH-R Ab (Stim)], which are found in autoimmune hyperthyroidism (Graves disease) for autoantibodies that bind to the TSH receptor and inhibit the activity of TSH [TSH-R Ab (block)]. The latter antibodies are found in patients with severe hypothyroidism, autoimmune atrophic thyroiditis and some infants with neonatal hypothyroidism.

Self-regulation in thyroid cells

Thyroid cells have the ability to regulate their production in T4 and T3 regardless of TSH activity and depending on the amount of iodine available in the blood.

In the case of low levels of iodine in the blood, an overproduction of active T3 over the production of T4 is adversely affected. When, on the contrary, there is an excess of iodine, the iodine itself causes inhibition of intracellular transport to be associated with tyrosines. Large amounts also inhibit other thyroid hormone synthesis factors such as TSH synthesis and TSH-R Ab (stim) stimulatory autoantibodies to the TSH receptor.

However, inhibition of secretion of thyroid hormones from the excess iodine is retained because the thyroid adjusting function and secrete normal amounts of hormones.

<u>Regular adjustment by thyroid hormones</u>

Thyroid hormones T4 and T3 act on hypothalamic TRH and pituitary TSH by inhibiting their secretion. This action, which is potent, is an important factor in retrograde regulation that maintains thyroid secretion in physiological states at desirable levels. The mechanism of this regulation and its intensity is evidenced by the administration of T4 and T3 at doses slightly hyper physiological which cause a decrease in secretion and a decrease in TSH in the blood and in the case of slight glib sub-function which results in an immediate increase in TSH in the blood.

<u>The action of deiodinases</u>

The inhibitory action of thyroid hormones in the hypothalamus and the pituitary gland and other tissue activities is dependent on the integrity and activity of deiodinases which can increase the activity of T4 and T3 if they favor the conversion of T4 to T3 or reduce it if enhance the conversion of T4 to rT3.

Pituitary and hypothalamic deiodinases, as well as liver deiodinases and other tissues, play a direct role in the regulation of thyroid hormone activity and indirect effect on thyroid function via T4 → T3 or T4 → rT3 → TRH → TSH → thyroid.

Other regulatory factors

In addition to the above basic factors that regulate thyroid function, there are other factors that have not been identified. First, the neurotransmitters that stimulate and inhibit the secretion of TRH and the TRH pulse responsible for the excretion of TRH and the day-to-day rhythm of TRH. Second, growth factors and cytokines and their local action on the thyroid and the pituitary and / or the hypothalamus. Third, the immune system and the production of antibodies against the TSH-R receptor by B lymphocytes.

Chapter 6: Thyroid functions and immune system

The immune system has as its primary mission the defense of the organism against foreign invaders. For this function, however, the defensive mechanisms of the immune system have the greatest specificity to distinguish the foreign from the body.

The immune system consists of a network of collaborating cellular and chemical elements, just like the endocrine system with which there is close interaction. If the elements of the immune system do not have or lose the sensitivity or the ability to recognize the stimulus and treat it as a stranger, or if the message they receive, even the friendly one stimulates them, the autoimmune disease is characterized by mobilization of the immune system turns against the friendly message and its source for destruction.

Thyroid function is often affected by autoimmune reactions generated by thyroid antigen production recognized as foreign elements by the immune system resulting in the formation of stimulatory or inhibitory antibodies accompanied by similar important functions and morphological lesions of the gland.

<u>Cellular elements of the immune system</u>

The immune response to the body's defense involves many kinds of cells, the most important being T and B lymphocytes and macrophages. Cells of the reticuloendothelial system and neutrophils also have defense properties against foreign bodies.

T lymphocytes provide cellular immunity, while B lymphocytes produce antibodies, that is, specific proteins, immunoglobulins, which undertake immunity.

Immune system chemicals

The immune system employs a wide variety of substances, which have the role of either chemical or chemical messenger receptors. The latter class of receptors belonging to the immune system is characterized by a unique diversity which is necessary for the identification of thousands of foreign substances and which is different in each individual so that substances belonging to individuals of the same animal or other species are recognized as strangers.

The variety of these receptors is genetically derived from 3 groups of genes:

1. Genes of the major histocompatibility complex that is characterized as human leukocyte antigen (HLA) in humans. HLA-encoding genes are in series on the short strand of chromosome 6 occupying an area of 4,000,000bp in which more than 40 genes were isolated. HLA genes are distinguished in three categories, the first of which expresses three genes of HLA-A, HLA-B and HLA-C, which encode only the α-chain proteins found in the cell membrane of all cells. The second class encodes the pairs of α and β chains of proteins that are also found in the cell membrane and are HLA-DR, HLA-DP and HLA-DQ.

2. Genes encoding immunoglobulins (Ig) and T lymphocyte receptors (TCR). Genes encoding immunoglobulins (Ig) and lymphocyte T (TCR) receptors may have the only unique property of being composed of small DNA sequences being expressed, i.e. only exons, which during cell progression from the ancestral to the mature form joining each other without introns. That is, the cut-off is done in DNA and not in the resulting mRNA. Thus, a continuous sequence expressing certain amino acids, that are joined together randomly to form the RNA in order to express their final product, is formed. In this way a huge variety of immunoglobulins and T lymphocyte receptors are created that are different in each lymphocyte. The way immunoglobulins and TCR recognize the antigens differ. Both recognize a portion of the antigen molecule, called epitope. The epitope for Ig consists of a few amino acids (3-20) and is readily recognizable in the antigen molecule, whereas for TCR the epitopes are more complex and the most important are only recognized when they are joined to HLA molecules located on the surface of specific cells of the immune system.

3. Collaborative cell surface proteins. In addition to HLA, Ig proteins and TCR proteins, protein molecules involved in immune function in different ways are present on the cell surface. For example, the message is received by the receptors or leads the cells to their action targets or assists the cell adhesion. TCRs bind to a differentiation complex. It has been named because the presence of these proteins is associated with differentiation of T lymphocytes during their maturation, which have intracellular extensions and transmit the signal to the inside of the cell and enhance or differentiate the sensitivity of T lymphocytes. Two predominantly TCRs linked to CDR, TCR-CD4 and TCR-CD8 are distinguished. Proteins that help to bind the antigen to the receptors belong to the immunoglobulin superfamily and are essential elements of the immune response. These proteins belong to the integrins and selectins.

4. Cytokines. The function of the immune system is also assisted by cytokines produced by a variety of cells including cells of the immune system. Cytokines have a strong effect on the growth, differentiation and activation of cell function.

5. Antibodies. The B cell lymphocyte cell membrane immunoglobulins, when detached from the cell and enter the circulation, are the antibodies. The form of the immunoglobulin secreted as an antibody consists of 2 regions, that binds to the antigen and the constant heavy chain region bound to various molecules and is distinguished in 5 major groups of IgM, IgD, IgG, IgE, IgA called isotopes . Each lymphocyte produces a kind of Ig.

Thyroid antibodies

Lymphocytic thyroiditis and hyperthyroidism have been among the first cases in which an autoimmune reaction was detected by the presence of autoantibodies in the serum of the patients. The anti-thyroid antibodies found are 4 and of these 2: a) the anti-thyroglobulins and b) the second colloid antigen have extracellular origin and the other two; c) the anti-peroxidase antibodies; and d) TSH are derived from thyroid cells.

• Antithyroglobulin antibodies (anti-Tg)

Anti-thyroglobulin (anti-Tg or TgAb) antibodies are detected by various methods and physiological values vary according to the assay method to be reported by the laboratory. Anti-Tg are found elevated in 50-70% of patients with lymphocytic thyroiditis (Hashimoto) and less in hyperthyroidism.

• The second colloid antigen (CA2)

The CA2 antigen is of unknown structure and function.

• Peroxidase Antibodies (TPOAb)

Thyroid Peroxidase (TPO) is the microsomal antigen that was previously identified by various methods and was called MSAb. After the microsomal antibody is identified with the peroxidase the antibody is called TPOAb and the assay is done using purified peroxidase.

• Antibodies to the TSH receptor

The presence of antibodies against the TSH receptor was detected in 1956-1960 without their known nature. The antibody was then named LATS by the property it had to stimulate thyroid function for a longer time than TSH. These antibodies have been shown to be directed against the TSH receptor found in the thyroid cell membrane. Antibodies to the TSH receptor (TSH-R) have been found to be of two kinds: a) Stimulants [TSH-Rab (Stim) or TSAb] which stimulate the receptor and activate, like TSH, all stages of thyroid hormone genesis, causing hyperthyroidism and b) inhibitors [TSH-Rab (block) or TBIAb] that inhibit receptor activity resulting in thyroid cell deficiency. TSH-Rab (stim) antibodies stimulate the placenta and may cause hyperthyroidism in the neonate, but this is transient because the antibodies do not reproduce but are metabolized and disappear. Another thyroglobulin took the name TSI and was thought to stimulate the function of thyroid cells because they are associated with them, but it turned out to be non-specific and its action is questioned.

Chapter 7: Laboratory tests for diagnosis of diseases of thyroid

Laboratory Tests:
1. Thickening of the thyroid gland
2. Ultrasound (V / S): Ultrasound performed to control the anatomy of the thyroid gland, to determine the size, position and number of potential nodes and to investigate the presence of any suspected lymph nodes in the wider area of the neck.
3. CAT scan: CT or magnetic resonance imaging (MRI) is sometimes indicated when more information is needed but not part of the initial evaluation.
4. Thyroid scintigraphy: If a nodule is detected after palpation of the thyroid, a scintigraphy needs to be done. This test evaluates its functional status (whether or not it produces thyroid hormone). The doctor administers a radioactive isotope injected into the gland, which is taken to a different extent from the ozone. The greater the amount of isotope the tumor gets, the more likely it is to be benign. This test is safe and does not pose health risks.
5. Total thyroid scintigraphy for Ca thyroid test
6. Blood examinations of thyroid hormones: Blood tests for T3- T4- FT3- FT4- TSH- Anti Tg, Anti TPO, Tg, calcitonin, Anti-TSH antibodies in the blood.

7. Histological examinations (biopsy): The histological examination is done when there is a nodule in the Thyroid. With a fine needle, cells are sucked out of the Thyroid tumor, and this biopsy can provide information as to whether cancer is or not. FNA biopsies are often done with an ultrasound guidance to obtain nodular formation cells and not the other gland leakage. This test has an extremely high sensitivity to diagnosis. Positive for malignancy is absolute evidence of surgery. The negative for malignancy does not guarantee the patient 100% for no malignancy, often presents false negative results (20%)

Chapter 8: Disorders of Thyroid Function

Thyroid function displays disorders that may take the form of hypo-function or hypothyroidism and hyper-function or hyperthyroidism.

An individual state of thyroid function is the simple goiter, which is characterized by hyperplasia of the gland without hormone hyper-secretion and which can be considered as a malfunction.

Non-specific thyroid inflammation, thyroiditis, causes functional disorders of the gland.

Biological and clinical quirks also show thyroid cancer.

8.1 Hypothyroidism

Hypothyroidism is a clinical syndrome resulting from the lack of thyroid hormones, which in turn leads to a generalized slowdown in metabolic processes. Hypothyroidism in infants and children causes a significant slowdown in growth and development, with severe permanent consequences, including permanent deprivation. The onset of hyperthyroidism after adulthood causes generalized slowing down of the organism by depositing glycoaminoglycans in the interstitial cell spaces, especially in the skin and muscles. The symptoms of hypothyroidism in adults are largely reversible with treatment.

Reason and effect

Hypothyroidism can be classified as:

1. primary (thyroid insufficiency)
2. Secondary (due to lack of pituitary TSH)
3. tertiary (due to hypothalamic TRH deficiency)
4. peripheral resistance to thyroid hormone activity

Thyroid sub function that creates a characteristic appearance of the patient because of skin lesions is called myxedema. Some use this term only for severe cases of hypothyroidism with severe skin symptom.

Thyroid sub function, depending on the age involved, forms a particular clinical picture characterized as:

a. adult hypothyroidism
b. neonatal hypothyroidism
c. child hypothyroidism
d. senile hypothyroidism

Particular forms of hypothyroidism are:

e. Clinical hypothyroidism
f. Postpartum hypothyroidism

a. Adult hypothyroidism

Adult hypothyroidism is not a rare disease. Hypothyroidism is more common in women in the proportion of 4-9 to 1 and in the 40-60 age group. The intensity with which the symptoms of hypothyroidism occur in adults varies from the form of mild manifestations that are difficult to distinguish from the physiological state and remain for a long time undiagnosed to the form of the trauma with characteristic lesions. Symptoms are sometimes so slow and progressive that the transition from normal to pathological is not perceived by sufferers. Hypothyroidism can also be manifested mono-symptomatically by the prevalence of symptoms of an organ due to its sensitivity to the lack of thyroid hormones.

a.i. Rationale

In adults, thyroid deficiency is due to 4 recurrent categories:

1. in thyroidogenic condition such as chronic lymphocytic thyroiditis (Hashimoto's disease), deficiency after treatment of hypothyroidism with radioiodine or surgical and, more rarely, chronic or high iodine intake. The most common cause (over 90%) of thyroid dysfunction is chronic thyroiditis (HSC) or Hashimoto's disease, which is usually accompanied by thyroid swelling but may have caused atrophy in the gland. The latter case is characterized as idiopathic thyroid atrophy. During CHL, the autoimmune reaction causes thyroid cell destruction and lymphocytic infiltration of the gland. Patients' serum contains antithyroid antibodies in various titers. Hypothyroidism after gland damage is often seen in the treatment of hyperthyroidism with radioactive iodine. The frequency of hypothyroidism is significant from the first year after treatment and progressively increases in the following years to reach over 50% within 10 years. The surgical treatment of hyperthyroidism, in which subtype thyroidectomy occurs, also involves the occurrence of hypothyroidism in a significant percentage (10-30%) and sometimes many years after surgery. The frequent presence in hyperthyroidism and TSH-RAB (Block) inhibitory antibodies favors the postoperative appearance of hypothyroidism. Rarely, the same happens during the surgery of a simple goiter, due to removal of a large part of the gland and destruction of the remainder. Acute thyroiditis can also result in permanent hypothyroidism. In rare cases, the expiration of a large amount of iodine in the form of a medicine for certain conditions (rheumatic diseases, bronchial diseases) and for a long period of time (months or years) causes hypothyroidism due to inhibition of thyroid hormone synthesis. It is believed that in these cases there is a slight enzyme disorder in the thyroid that is exacerbated by taking iodine preparations.

2. In a hypophysiogenic cause, such as in the pituitary insufficiency due to adenoma development or surgery. Diseases of the pituitary and hypothalamus can also cause thyroid atrophy and secondary hypothyroidism in adults due to non-secretion of TSH. The most common cause of secondary hypothyroidism is pituitary adenomas and surgical procedures in the pituitary gland.

3. Rarely in possible hypothalamic dysfunction. Very rare thyroid dysfunction may be due to hypothalamic lesion. In this case, it is called tertiary hypothyroidism, the functioning of thyroid cells is normal, as evidenced by the hypothalamic TRH response.

4. Extremely rare in peripheral resistance to thyroid hormone action. Thyroid hormone resistance syndrome is characterized by goiter, increased thyroid hormone (T4 and T3), slightly elevated or normal TSH, which is normally found in TRH and is not inhibited or partially inhibited by T3 and most of the metabolic hyper secretion of T4 and T3.

All of the above changes are interpreted to be due to the resistance of tissues including thyroid stimulating cells to the action of T4 and T3. The damage in some individuals has been detected in the thyroid hormone receptor gene (TR gene).

The condition is hereditary and occurs with varying intensity and symptomatology among the various members of the family of sufferers. Symptoms may be hyperthyroid or rarely hypothyroidism, and most of the time there is only a goiter with no apparent catabolic disorder. The diversity of events is attributed to the different response or resistance of the various tissues to thyroid hormones. There are even cases that present at the same time hyperthyroidism.

The frequency of the syndrome does not appear to be too small as more than 600 cases have been reported.

a.ii. Pathological physiology

The lack of thyroid hormones explains the clinical and biological manifestations of hypothyroidism. The variety of symptoms and involvement in the hypothyroid status of most organs and tissues underline the great biological importance of thyroid hormones for the body.

The major disorder of hypothyroidism is the slowing down of essential intracellular functions that require energy, such as oxygen consumption by mitochondria. The reduction in energy consumption results in hypo-metabolism that is clinically evident from low basal metabolism, low body temperature and abnormalities in the functioning of various organs.

Synthesis and in particular degradation of fats slows down in hypothyroidism, resulting in hypercholesterolemia and hypertriglyceridemia and the relative increase in β-lipoproteins. The synthesis and degradation of albumins and especially albumin is also slow. Absorption of glucose from the gastrointestinal tract and its peripheral use is reduced.

A slow pace and a small pulse volume are observed in the heart, resulting in a reduction in cardiac output. The size of the heart is increased due to exudate present in the pericardium and myocardial lesions. The electrograph has low spikes and often displays abnormalities of the T-pattern.

Kidney function is impaired due to decreased glomerular filtration and reabsorption and discharge capacity of the urinary tubules.

The gastrointestinal system displays muscle hypotonia and secretory subfunction.

The metabolic functions of the brain are significantly affected by hypothyroidism. The disorder of brain function is perceived by mental, sensory and motor disorders and by lesions of the electroencephalogram.

Skeletal muscles show an increase in their volume and slowness in contraction and relaxation. The muscles of the limbs and the tongue are affected more often. Hypertrophy and contractile abnormalities create stiffness in the muscles and difficulties in the movements and joint. Tendon reflexes for the same reasons become slow.

Finally, skin has accumulated in the connective tissue, around the vessels and near its components, such as mucopolysaccharides, hyaluronic acid, chondroitin sulfate. These substances, together with sodium retention in the extracellular space, create the edematous condition in hypothyroidism.

a.iii. Symptomology

Hypothyroidism when presented with complete symptomatology is characterized by: 1. Skin lesions, 2. Hypothermia, 3. Muscular weakness, 4. Gastrointestinal disorders, 5. Psycho-mental disorders, 6. Bradycardia, 7. Slowness of speech and voice of the voice, 8. the hearing loss.

1. skin lesions are the most specific and characteristic of the hypothyroidism symptom and therefore helps diagnose. The skin is dry, of low temperature, rough, invisible, wrinkled and shows hyperkeratosis at friction points. The mucous membranes are filtered, resulting in increased tongue volume, thickening of the vocal cords and ectopic trumpet. The hairs are fragile, rough, dry, easily falling, resulting in thinning of hair, eyebrows, armpit hair. Nails are brittle, thick and show streaks. In the face the skin lesions create a myxedematic mask, characterized by: a. Filtered eyelids, which leave a small bluff slit, b. Thick lips and ears, c. Thick and wide nose, d. The thinning of the hair in the eyebrows, especially in their tail (point of the eyebrow tail), e. Deep wrinkles of the face, g. the filtered, but sometimes cyanotic, faces, great tongue, h. the abject expression. The throat is thick due to the infiltration of the skin. The hands of the hypothyroid patient are square with cylindrical fingers, which are cold, dry, have a rough touch, and are filtered by the dorsal and pale palmar surface. The roughness of the skin, and especially its hyperkeratosis, is perceived in the elbows and knees.

2. Hypothermia is manifested by low body temperature and poor cold tolerance. Sensitivity to cold is very characteristic and intense in hypothyroid and causes patients to dress more and to seek a warm environment.

3. Muscular weakness is common and sometimes occurs in the form of myopathy. There is also stiffness of the muscles that is particularly pronounced in finger movements in the morning during awakening. The muscles may be hypertrophic especially in the hands and legs. Typical is the slow relaxation of the muscles during the release of the reflexes.

4. Gastrointestinal disorders manifest with persistence and intense constipation. Reduction of appetite, indigestion, atony and bloating of the intestines are often phenomena. Despite the decrease in appetite the weight remains normal or slightly increased. Significant, however, obesity is rarely seen in hypothyroidism.

5. Psycho-mental disorders are common. They consist of cold-headedness, decreased attention and interest in the environment, slowness of association and memory disturbances. The emotional site is diminished. Pure psychotic events are not uncommon. At the same time, the movements of the sufferer are slow and uncommon.

6. Bradycardia, dullness of heart tones and in advanced states, heart failure are seen from the cardiovascular system.

7. Speech is slow and sticky due to muscle stiffness. The voice is hoarse and her tone low.

8. Acoustic capacity is reduced due acoustic nerve damage.

a.iv. Laboratory findings

The basic and necessary finding in hypothyroidism is the low values of thyroid hormones in the blood. A very sensitive indicator of low thyroid hormone levels is the increase in TSH, which may reveal a hypothyroid disorder if the T4 and T3 values are marginal. The total thyroxine value is less than 50 ng / ml and T3 of 0.7 ng / ml. Similar are the values of free T4 and free T3. TSH, which normally ranges from 0.5 and 5 μUU / ml, is above 15 μUU / ml and can reach 150 μUU / ml. The retention of radioactive iodine by the thyroid rarely exceeds 10% of the dose and does not increase further after stimulation with TSH. Often in the blood of the hypothyroid, there are high titers of anti-thyroid antibodies which reveal the immune defect of the gland. In the blood, too, cholesterol is increased and can reach values up to 450-600 mg / 100ml. Anemia is present in a large proportion of patients. The electrocardiogram exhibits a slowing of the rate and a reduction in the height of the fields, which may be so characteristic that hypothyroidism is suspected by the cardiologist. Chest X-ray reveals a large cardiac shadow due to excretion of the pericardium.

a.v. Diagnosis

Hypothyroidism when presented with the comprehensive and intense symptomatology described is easily diagnosed clinically.

Difficulties arise in 2 cases: a. When the onset of symptoms occurs at a slow pace and their intensity is low so that the transition from normal to pathological is not evident, b. When some symptoms appear unilaterally in a bold form to overshadow other events, to draw attention to the organ from which they originate and to develop a disease of that organ.

The gradual establishment of symptoms is common in hypothyroidism and is the cause of the inadequate diagnosis of the disease. The clinical picture before completing symptomatology is not typical and requires a great deal of diagnostic ability from part of a physician to distinguish hypothyroid symptoms when they appear in a mild form and separate them from common events. Careful analysis of the symptoms and clinical examination and evaluation of the changes that occurred to the patient in relation to his or hers previous condition lead most of the time to the correct diagnosis. When there are doubts, the laboratory tests solve the problem.

The occurrence of hypothyroidism with noisy symptomatology by an organ or system can also mislead the diagnosis.

The mental manifestations of hypothyroidism may take the form of acute or chronic psychosis, the phenomena of which distract attention and lead the patient to neurological clinics for the treatment of mental illness.

The invasion of the muscular system can be so intense as to be a muscular disease.

Anemia, when important, leads to a misdiagnosis of hematologic disease and unnecessary therapies, because the hematological image is corrected by the treatment of hypothyroidism.

Hypotension and underactive bowel and gallbladder, along with anorexia, create the impression of cholecystitis or liver disease and remove thought from hypothyroidism.

In all the above cases it is necessary to differentiate hypothyroidism from the diseases of the organs presenting the pathological manifestations. The diagnosis will be based on the search for the remaining symptoms of hypothyroidism and will be confirmed in laboratory.

a.vi. Treatment

The treatment of hypothyroidism is the administration of thyroid hormones in substitution doses. It is preferred to administer thyroxine, due to its conversion to T3.

Treatment follows a number of rules, the most basic of which is to start in small doses and progressively increase them to maintenance doses.

The beneficial effect of treatment is quick. Within a few days the edematous infiltration begins to sub serve, especially on the face, the skin is exfoliated and becomes softer and warmer, the patient feels that he recovers strength and begins to emerge from previous inertia and apathy. At the same time it loses weight, shows increased diuresis and increased energy.

Within a few weeks blood cholesterol decreases, the electrocardiogram improves and the other functions are restored so that within 2-3 months the patient is completely healthy.

Hypothyroid patients are particularly susceptible to thyroid hormones. Overdose or abrupt increase may cause extraordinary contractions, headache, dyspnoea, anxiety, and anginal seizures. If side effects occur, treatment is discontinued for several days and repeated in smaller doses.

b. Neonatal hypothyroidism

Hypothyroidism that occurs in childhood has a serious impact on the developing organism and a heavy prognosis for the psycho-social development and physical development of the child, since it is not addressed in time. The heavy form of congenital hypothyroidism accompanied by great mental retardation is also called cretinism (the term is not used).

At birth and neonatal age the onset of hypothyroidism requires rapid diagnosis and immediate treatment to prevent permanent damage.

The risks of lack of thyroid hormones are mainly related to cerebral functions, as the absence of the brain in the perinatal period is observed, as brain development is supplemented by 70% in the first 2 years after birth.

In addition, in neonatal hypothyroidism, gland deficiency is usually large or even complete, and for this the manifestations of the disease are premature and the need for rapid treatment.

However, most cases of neonatal hypothyroidism remain undiagnosed or are diagnosed late with the result that patients have unresolved brain damage and are a major problem for their families, with severe medical and social consequences.

In the previous states, the risk of neonatal hypothyroidism is addressed by detecting disease in all newborns. The detection of hypothyroidism is done by measuring in the blood of THS and thyroid hormones. Every newborn on the fifth day of birth is taken from the heel drop of blood. This drop determines TSH or T4 or both. The incidence of neonatal hypothyroidism in Greece is 1 in every 4-5,000 births.

b.i. Rationale

The main cause of neonatal hypothyroidism is anatomical abnormalities of the gland. More rarely, the condition is due to fetal thyroid injury or to an enzyme disorder of hormone genesis.

The anatomical anomalies of the thyroid can be: a. complete lack of the gland (atherosclerosis), b. ectopia, c. hypoplasia, d. dyspepsia of the thyroid.

The administration of therapeutic radioactive iodine during pregnancy or, more rarely, the ingestion of large amounts of iodine or anti-thyroid medication, may cause damage to the function of the fetal thyroid and the occurrence of hypothyroidism after birth.

Hormonal disorders are rarely so severe as to cause a significant reduction in thyroid hormone and hypothyroidism during the neonatal period.

b.ii. Symptomology

Hypothyroid disease is not usually evident at birth due to the circulation of even limited, even limited, maternal thyroid hormones in the fetus. Depending on the severity of the deficiency, however, the symptoms appear. Birth weight is usually large (> 4,000g), while the length of the newborn is moderate.

The main clinical events in the first weeks come from the gastrointestinal tract, respiratory system, psychomotor growth and skin.

The gastrointestinal system has a long and persistent constipation and is accompanied by abdominal and umbilical enlargement. The appetite is small, the baby is reluctant to breastfeed, the tongue is large and sometimes protrudes from the mouth and feeding becomes difficult. Normal neonatal jaundice is longer than normal.

Respiratory disorders include respiratory distress and episodes of cyanosis or drowning especially during pregnancy.

The psychomotor development of the newborn is pathological. The child is unusually calm, immobile, sleeping continuously, his screaming is rare and his voice hoarse and deep.

The skin is dry, cold, dense, amber, with cyanogenic areas.

Over the course of months, two clinical events have become particularly prominent:

• The slowdown in psychomotor growth. The infant does not smile, does not hold his head, does not sit, does not show the first teeth, nor does it show closure of the skull springs at defined ages. At the same time it is environmentally friendly, inert and indifferent to toys.

• The inhibition of physical development. There is a slowing of the increase in length and less of the weight increase.

At the same time hypothermia, bradycardia is observed and the hypothyroid emerges.

The clinical picture of neonatal and infant hypothyroidism depends on the severity of the lesion.

b.iii. Laboratory findings and diagnosis

The diagnosis of neonatal hypothyroidism is based on finding low thyroid hormone (T4 and T3) and high TSH values. Bone X-ray offers valuable information to neonatal and childhood hypothyroidism. The radiography shows: a. the presence of the osteogenic nuclei, b. the existence of physical dysgenesis.

1. Osteonecrosis occurs at a defined age. Their appearance depends on thyroid hormones Thyroid deficiency always results in a delay in the appearance of osteoporotic nuclei, so that from the study of nuclei that exist and that have not yet appeared, it is possible to place, not only, the diagnosis of hypothyroidism but to determine the possible time of installation.

2. Painful dysgenesis consists of the fragmentation of the pineal gland because it is ossified in an abnormal and inhomogeneous manner. Painful dysgenesis is a hallmark of hypothyroidism.

At birth in normal children there are knee bone nuclei (femur and tibia) formed from the 8th fetal month and the kernel bone of the tarsus, which appears just before birth. In neonatal hypothyroidism the above nuclei are absent. If they exist and show epiphyseal dysgenesis, it is concluded that the hypothyroid status was established a few weeks prior to birth. Cholesterol is elevated in blood in a large proportion of patients.

When the above laboratory methods are not accessible, the diagnosis is based on the clinical picture and is confirmed by the therapeutic criterion, the rapid change of the image and the improvement of the condition under the effect of the treatment.

b.iv. Treatment

Treatment is easy and simple and consists in administering thyrexin at doses initially small that will increase incrementally to maintenance doses. The maintenance dose is determined by controlling the TSH value, which should return to normal levels. The prognosis if treatment begins early after birth is excellent. Otherwise, the risk of brain damage is high.

c. Child hypothyroidism

Childhood hypothyroidism is either congenital, but light in order to manifest itself in older age or acquired due to gland damage that occurred after birth. Child hypothyroidism differs from neonatal in: a. the frequency of the different reasons, b. clinical events that predominate in every form.

c.i. Rationale

The etiology of the disease in childhood is a) thyroid gynecomastia (2/3 of cases); b) idiopathic deficiency; c) enzymatic disorders of hormone genesis; and d) use of broncho-constrictors.

- The most common cause of hypothyroidism in children is the ectopic position of the thyroid. The ectopic gland is in the middle line at some point in the course of its fetal migration. Mostly, it is at the root of the thyroid and the normal position of the thyroid.
- The automatic appearance of hypothyroidism without apparent cause (idiopathic) resembles the corresponding adult status.
- Enzymatic disorders of hormone genesis that cause thyroid deficiency are rare, familial, and have hereditary features. These abnormalities are usually accompanied by a simple goiter and etiology. In these cases, glandular hyperplasia is not sufficient to compensate for enzyme damage and the amount of thyroid hormone secreted is reduced, resulting in the appearance of, in addition to the goiter and points of hypothyroidism. The size of the goiter does not prejudge the existence of sub-operation.
- The use of broncho-constrictors in childhood is a rare cause of hypothyroidism.

c.ii. Symptomology

The most characteristic manifestations of child hypothyroidism are the delay of physical growth and morphological manifestations. Regular growth rates exclude hypothyroidism, unless it is very recent. Growth inhibition or deceleration of growth is made early by parents. At the same time morphological changes are observed. The head is large, the base of the nose wide, the trunk of the normal size, and the limbs close. The morphological alterations above form a characteristic appearance of the patient. At the same time there are other manifestations of hypothyroidism. Skin lesions, constipation, poor cold tolerance, almost always accompany child hypothyroidism, varying in intensity, depending on the severity of the deficiency. Intellectual retardation may be mild or not apparent in preschool age and become apparent only when the patient starts school and compares with his classmates.

c.iii. Laboratory findings and diagnosis

The diagnosis of hypothyroid status in childhood, which can be manifested by mild symptomatology, is done by measuring thyroid hormones and blood TSH. In disputed cases, with T4, T3 and TSH limit values, the TRH assay reveals a high TSH stimulus. Radiological testing detects bone osteoarthritis and epinephrine dysgenesis and determines the degree of bone maturation. This calculates the patient's bone age, which is always delayed. Radioisotope testing allows for the location, size and functional capacity of the thyroid.

c.iv. Treatment

The treatment is done with the administration of thyroxine and is aimed at restoring: (a) Euthyroidism; (b) Normal Growth Rate. The treatment continues for life, without interruption. The dose ranges between 100-150 μg L thyroxine and the efficacy is controlled by measuring blood TSH. During treatment, the bone age of the patient should be checked to ensure hormonal growth of the body and maturation of the skeleton. The final height of the patients depends on the age at which the treatment starts and on the initial short-sightedness. If the diagnosis is made early and treatment is started at an early age, the stature of the patients when they become adults, it is normal. The puberty in hypothyroid children receiving regular treatment occurs naturally evolve. Normal also is their reproductive capacity when they become adults.

d. Senile hypothyroidism

The incidence of disease after the 60th year is not small. According to statistics it is 0.5-6% for clinically evident hypothyroidism and up to 4-15% for the subclinical. In women the incidence after 75 years of age increases by 1.3% per year. The most common cause of hypothyroidism in the elderly is autoimmune thyroiditis with goiter or atrophic thyroiditis.

The diagnosis is usually performed in severe forms only with complete symptomatology. Treatment also has problems due to the age of the sufferers.

The difficulty of detecting hypothyroidic conditions in the elderly is due to the fact that the main manifestations of the disease are perceived as a consequence of old age.

Thus, the skin of the elderly has lost its turgidity, is pale and often cold due to poor circulation. Poor tolerance of cold is common in elders. Easy fatigue is almost rule because of old age. Constipation is plagued by older ages and the decline in psycho-functional functions is a common phenomenon in old age.

Within this image, which is the physiological state of most elderly people, the detection of hypothyroidal elements requires great diagnostic sensitivity. For this reason, recourse to the laboratory is more necessary in the older age and the diagnosis is mainly based on the results of the laboratory tests.

Treatment of senile hypothyroidism should be treated with caution. The cardiovascular system, which is aging due to old age, has also suffered from the harmful effects of hypothyroidism, usually for a long time, due to delayed diagnosis. Atherosclerosis is more common in inferior hypothyroid. The heart, however, responds to the needs of the body, because they are scarce because of reduced metabolism, on the other hand because physical activity is reduced.

During treatment, the increase in metabolic processes and the activity of the sufferer entails a heavy burden on the circulatory needs, in which the heart is difficult to respond. For this reason, there is a risk of angina or heart failure during treatment. Doses of thyroxine should initially be small, be increased slowly and staggered, and the maintenance dose should be set to less than normal, depending on the patient's reaction and tolerability.

e. Subclinical hypothyroidism

Elevated TSH values with normal T3 and T4 values are observed in many cases. People with normal thyroid hormone levels and lack of obvious symptoms in combination with increased TSH, which means reduced thyroid hormone activity, at least at the pituitary level, are thought to have subclinical hypothyroidism. The incidence of this condition in the general population is not small and increases in the elderly. The increased tendency for medical testing, which usually involves measuring thyroid hormones, reveals more and more often the hormonal abnormalities of subclinical hypothyroidism, especially in the elderly and creates diagnostic and therapeutic problems.

The most common cause of subclinical hypothyroidism is chronic thyroiditis, as predicted by the frequent coexistence of antithyroid antibodies and the previous hyperthyroidism being treated.

Clinical hypothyroidism accompanied by high titers of anti-thyroid antibodies should be treated with substitution therapy. In subclinical hypothyroidism without antithyroid antibodies, treatment or monitoring will depend on the level of TSH, T4 and T3, the age and general condition of the patients and will be personalized.

f. Postpartum hypothyroidism

Postpartum is frequent occurrence of autoimmune thyroiditis. Its incidence is estimated to be about 5-6% of women, many of whom show marked symptoms of hypothyroidism or rarely hyperthyroidism, usually 3-6 months postpartum.

Hypothyroidism is most of the time transient, and this is another reason why this condition remains undetected despite the relatively high incidence.

The condition is attributed to an exacerbation of autoimmune disease that has been suppressed like all immune responses during pregnancy: women with an individual or family history of autoimmune disease or high titers of antithyroid antibodies are prone to postpartum thyroiditis and hypothyroidism. The condition is exacerbated after each parturition and may result in permanent hypothyroidism. Hypothyroidism may also occur in the form manifested by hypothyroid symptoms.

Diagnosis requires medical attention and diagnosis, because symptoms are attributable to anxiety, depression, anemia and other causes. Diagnosis is easily confirmed by measuring thyroid hormones and treating and relieving patients is also easy. Because of the urgency of hypothyroidism after childbirth, treatment should be interrupted and thyroid function controlled.

g. Hypophysiogenic (secondary) hypothyroidism

Thyroid deficiency can be caused by pituitary damage and lack of secretion of thyroid stimulating hormone. In most cases, it is a multiple pituitary insufficiency. Individual lack of TSH is very rare. Generalized pituitary damage is mimicked as hypothyroidism when the manifestations of thyroid deficiency are intense and dominate the clinical picture overlapping the other symptoms. Attention to these cases is directed at thyroid, recognition of pituitary episode is of great importance for treatment and prognosis. The diagnosis will be based on 2 points: (a) the finding of pituitary damage; and (b) the discovery of characteristic laboratory findings of hypophysiogenic hypothyroidism.

• Pituitary insufficiency is documented by historical, clinical symptoms and laboratory findings. Symptoms of pituitary adenoma (particularly headache and ophthalmological disorders) particularly evident when they are hormone-secreted and deficiency manifestations of other peripheral glands (gonads, adrenal glands) or history of childbearing under anemia (Sheehan syndrome) of a pituitary insufficiency, which is easily confirmed in laboratory.

• The distinctive feature of pituitary hypothyroidism is low blood TSH, which exists alongside low thyroid hormones, as opposed to thyroidogenic primary hypothyroidism, where TSH is very high. Also, in hypophysiogenic hypothyroidism, TSH does not respond to TRH administration.

There are, however, rare cases of secondary hypothyroidism, in which TSH is found in the blood at normal levels and the response to TRH administration is normal. In these cases, the lesion is located in the hypothalamus and is due to a lack or reduced secretion of TRH, which causes functional deficiency of TSH secretion, resulting in thyroid dysfunction. This form is called hypothalamic or tertiary hypothyroidism.

Anti-thyroid antibodies, which are so common in primary hypothyroidism, are rarely found in the hypophysiogenic. Cholesterol is also less and less frequently elevated.

The manifestations of hypo-pharyngeal hypothyroidism differ from the primary in some details. The skin is cold but thinner and less infiltrated. Head hair is also thinner. The tongue is visibly swollen. There is discoloration of the nipples.

When treating hypo-pharyngeal hypothyroidism, the primary disease that caused pituitary insufficiency (e.g. adenoma) and the functional status of the peripheral glands, especially the adrenal glands, should be considered. When there is no information on adrenal function, treatment begins with cortisol for prophylaxis of an acute adrenal insufficiency, which is more easily released when the patient leaves the hypothyroid disorder. A few days later, normal thyroxine therapy begins.

h. Myxedema coma

Myxedema coma is called the extreme state of hypothyroidism in which the bodily and cerebral functions of the body are reduced to the extent that the patient falls into coma.

Myxedema coma appears in neglected and undiagnosed conditions of hypothyroidism, in elderly people usually, due to the diagnostic function of the disease in old age. Most cases involve women aged 60-70 years.

Emotional factors of the coma are infections (especially pneumonia), exposure to cold (more frequent in winter), surgical procedures, wounds, psychosocial use. The coma occurs abruptly or after a dormant stage.

h.i. Symptomology

The status is characterized by:

1. the image of hypothyroidism: the hypothyroid image is typical because there are all symptoms of the disease and to a high degree. Particularly evident is the facial mask, the skin and hair lesions, the abdomen.

2. the characters of the coma: Coma is deep, without processes, with reduction or elimination of reflexes. Neurological manifestations are not uncommon: convulsions, muscle stiffness, pyramidal signs.

3. hypothermia: Hypothermia is the hallmark of the myxedemic coma. Body temperature may be below 30°, skin is frozen and dry. Finding normal temperature should suspect an infection.

4. bradycardia: Bradycardia is important and is accompanied by low patterns in the electrocardiogram.

5. breathlessness, which is interrupted by insomnia, is also characteristic.

h.ii. Diagnosis

The diagnosis of coma should be done clinically because laboratory confirmation by measuring thyroid hormones and TSH requires a precious time that cannot be lost. Differential diagnosis will be made by neurological coma with no hypothyroid manifestations and pituitary coma, which exhibits, in addition to hypothyroidism, extensive adrenal insufficiency and severe hypoglycemia.

h.iii. Treatment

Treatment should be immediate and intensive. Intravenously, 300-400 μg of thyroxine is administered once or 25-100 μg T3 every 12 hours. Cortisone (100-300 mg daily) is administered intravenously and electrolyte disturbances and hypoglycaemia are treated accordingly. Respiratory function is enhanced by the administration of oxygen or mechanical ventilator. Reheating the patient with warm pads becomes progressive to avoid circulatory shock. Despite the therapeutic efforts, the mortality of myxedemic coma is great.

8.2 Hyperthyroidism

Hyperthyroidism is called the condition resulting from the overproduction of thyroid hormones. The large production of thyroid hormones can be due either to hyper-function and hyper-secretion of the entire thyroid gland, so we have diffuse toxic goiter or Basedow's disease or Graves's disease, or over-function of a part of the gland in which an autonomic toxic adenoma has developed. These two form hyperthyroidism to which most of the cases belong. A third form of hyperthyroidism, the polyose toxic goiter is mainly observed in the elderly. It is characterized by the presence of autonomic secretory nodes and behaves like the single autonomous toxic adenoma. Underlying thyroiditis may also present at its initial stage of hyperthyroidism by the intense release of thyroid hormones caused by inflammation of the gland. Hyperthyroidism is transient but can cause diagnostic problems especially when thyroiditis is asymptomatic or appears with mild symptoms.

a. Diffuse toxic goiter (Basedow's Disease or Graves's Disease)

Hyper-operation and simultaneous hyperplasia of the entire gland resulting in hyper-secretion of thyroid hormones is the most common form of hyperthyroidism. It affects all ages with a higher incidence age range of 20-40 years.

a.i. Rationale

Investigation of the cause has gone through many stages. The inherited incidence of the thyroid physiological initiator of TSH was found to be inaccurate because TSH is not elevated in hyperthyroidism but is under strong inhibition to an extent that cannot be stimulated by hypothalamic TRH. The discovery in 1956 of a serum immunoglobulin, which exhibits stimulatory activity in thyroid cell function, and thus etiology has been shifted to the immune system. This immunoglobulin was named LATS (long acting thyroid stimulator) because it had the characteristic that its action was more prolonged than TSH. LATS belong to IgC globules, are found in the serum of many but not all of the hyperthyroid, but also in non-hyperthyroid individuals. This is an obstacle to accepting as a factor in the disease. Other immunoglobulins that exhibit thyroid stimulating activity were called TSI (thyroid stimulating immynoglobulins). In 1990, LANS was found to be an antibody produced by the TSH receptor in thyroid cells which acted as an antigen and was named TSH-RAb since then and was considered the major agent of hyperthyroidism and the disease is a part of the autoimmune diseases of the body. TSH-RAb binds to the TSH receptor and activates it, resulting in stimulation of all thyroid cell functions and hyper-secretion of thyroid hormones. In addition to the immune factor in the manifestation of hyperthyroidism, heredity, emotions, high iodine levels play a role. The hereditary factor is underlined by the presence of family history and other cases of hyperthyroidism, which are not uncommon, or the presence of thyroiditis, which is more common. Reinforcement is the existence of some specific antigens of the HLA system in relation to the general population. Hyperthyroidism has an increased incidence of HLA-B8 and HLA-DR3. Also, in the disease there are intense emotional states, due to the suppression of the immune system observed by the emotional stress that favors the appearance of hyperthyroidism. Taking large amounts of iodine may be a cause of hyperthyroidism. This condition is known as Jod-Basedow and is mainly seen in people with iodopenic goiter, who prophylactically take iodine or iodinated supplements. Infections may still be an elicitor of the disease or recurrence.

a.ii. Pathological physiology

In hyperthyroidism all thyroid functions are performed at an increased rate. Iodine uptake is faster and longer. The synthesis of thyroid hormones and their release is rapid. At the same time, glandular hyperplasia increases the hormone mass, while hyperemia facilitates the intake of raw materials and better supports metabolic exchange and thus contributes to increased hormonal production.

Thyroid hormones secreted in increased amount disappear faster than circulation and are found in the blood in free and active form at a higher proportion than normal.

This creates a state of excess thyroid hormone in the body that interprets most of the symptoms of the disease. The main ones, such as tachycardia, tremor, sweating, are pure adrenergic effects, and their manifestation is believed to be due to the increase in the number and sensitivity of adrenergic receptors by thyroid hormones. The administration of β-receptor blockers substantially eliminates or reduces these symptoms.

Two of the symptoms are due to the hyper-secretion of thyroid hormones: 1. exorbitant, due to the prolapse of the bulb from the increase in the backbone tissue volume, and 2. the local myxedema. Administration of thyroid hormones never causes these symptoms and therefore their pathogenicity is due to immune disorders of the disease. In the eyelid, the conjunctival nerve tissue increases and concentration of large amounts of mucopolysaccharides is observed. The muscles are poisoned and filtered by lymphocytes and plasma cells. The whole histological image reminds of autoimmune damage, which is confirmed by the finding that ophthalmic muscles bind specific anti-thyroglobulin antibodies and that retrotrobic tissue is a source of lymphocyte sensitizing antigen production.

a.iii.Symptomology

Hyperthyroidism is manifested by five-way symptoms:

• Bulging eyeball, it is a great diagnostic as it is easily understood and does not appear in many other conditions. Ejaculation is due to 2 changes in the eyes:

1. Contraction of the upper eyelid due to muscular hypertonia. Normally, the upper eyelid in the horizontal eye covers the iris respectively at the 10th and 12th hour. In hyperthyroidism due to contraction, part of the hard between the upper eyelid and the iris appears.

2. Incidence of the bulb, which is visible mainly from the side and is due to the retroviral tissue infiltration. In some cases, eyelid edema is also observed.

The combination of these two elements and in particular the contraction of the upper eyelid causes a characteristic luminous look or even expression of terror. Eyelid convergence is not common and is incomplete and this exposes the eye to the risk of inflammation or corneal ulceration. Upper eyelid contraction is best understood when the eye moves downwards because the eyelid follows slowly and thus appears with a larger portion of the hard above the pupil (Graefe point). Hemorrhagic and edematous conjunctivitis is common in hyperthyroid ejaculomas as well as muscle weakness, which causes diplopia. Ophthalmic symptoms are mainly somatic but not symmetrical. Often their onset is asynchronous and the changes in one eye are more pronounced.

- The goiter is usually of moderate size and is noticeable when palpable. The gland in most cases is diffusely swollen and the composition of the semi-dry or rubber. Vascularity is large and palpation can be found in the upper part of the lobes or more often at the hearing.
- Tachycardia is an important element of hyperthyroidism. It is permanent and is observed during calm, but it increases in emotions. The pulse ranges from 100 to 120 puffs per minute. Heartbeat pulses are strong and the arteries vibrate intensely. During the muscular effort the heart rate increases and shows dyspnea. Extreme contractions or seizures of tachycardia are common, especially in people over 40 years of age. Atrial fibrillation and absolute arrhythmia are not rare in elderly patients and may occur prematurely in younger individuals.
- Terror is mainly related to the limbs and is continuous, thin, fast and independent of will. Hand tremors have difficulty writing and fine work.

- Weight loss is typical. The patient may lose within a few weeks several pounds despite regular food intake and appetite preservation.
- Muscle weakness is common in hyperthyroidism and may take the form of myopathy. It manifests as easy fatigue in the people or climbing a ladder.
- Thermophobia consists in the inaccessibility of the warm environment. In summer, patients suffer from heat and in winter they dress lightly. At night they are covered with light covers. The thermophobia is due to vasodilatation, increased heat dissipation and increased body temperature. Thin sweat covers the body of sufferers and sweating becomes intense in the slightest effort. Characteristic are the warm, wet hands of the hyperthyroid.
- Hyperthyroid patients often experience nervousness, irritability, hyperactivity and emotionality. Patients cannot calm down, they are in constant movement, they are anxious, they react strongly to the stimuli, their movements are spasmodic, they are unstable emotionally, and they easily break into sobs. Their sleep is normal. Bowel hyperactivity is observed in a proportion of patients and is manifested by frequent emptyings that rarely take the form of diarrhea. In a small percentage of patients, local myxedema is observed in the lower extremities.
- The above symptoms usually occur at the same time and progressively deteriorate, making it difficult to accurately determine the onset of the disease. In other cases the symptoms manifest asynchronously and with different intensity. Sudden onset of disease with complete and intense symptoms is not uncommon.

a.iv. Laboratory findings

In hyperthyroidism, thyroid hormones are found in the blood increased. The radioimmunoassay of thyroxine gives values above 120 ng / ml (or 154 nmol / L) and the T3 measurement above 2.2 ng / ml (or 3.38 nmol / L). Free T4 and T3 are significantly elevated. The T3RU test is over 35%. This test reveals the amount of thyroid hormone-binding plasma proteins (TBG) and the number of binding sites that have been blocked. If there is little TBG or large amounts of endogenous thyroxine and T3, T3RU gives higher values, as in the case of hyperthyroidism.

The characteristic but laboratory finding of hyperthyroidism is suppression of TSH, which is detected by modern methods of measuring the high sensitivity hormone. TSH is <0.1 µU / ml and in the early stages of the disease when T4 and T3 are elevated.

The radioiodine retention is high from the first 2-4 hours. Because of the rapid production and release of thyroid hormones, retention at 24 hours is usually lower than that of the 3rd hour. High retention is not inhibited by T3 (T3 test) administration. The scintigraph shows no sign of anything. Even direct measurement of TSH and T3 and T4 is performed by radioimmunoassay.

a.v. Diagnosis

In most cases, the diagnosis of hyperthyroidism is based on the characteristic clinical picture and is only clinically confirmed. In most cases, both of the thyroid hormones are elevated, T3 is usually more than T4 and TSH is suppressed and this sets or confirms the diagnosis. When the increase in thyroid hormone is not high, low TSH or a lack of response to the TRH test is a strong indication of hyperthyroidism. In rare cases, only T3 (T3 hyperthyroidism) or, more rarely, only T4 (T4 hyperthyroidism) is elevated. Diagnosis of hyperthyroidism is difficult when the onset of symptoms is slow and progressive. In these cases the diagnostic difficulty lies in the separation of hyperthyroidism from neuronal manifestations accompanied by hypertonia of the neurological system, and they may experience tachycardia, tremor, weight loss and other thyroid overactive symptoms. Careful assessment of each event allows diagnosis most often, which is guaranteed by appropriate laboratory tests. Particularly difficult is the diagnosis of hyperthyroidism in the elderly. Mono-symptomatic manifestation of hyperthyroidism in the form of myopathy may disorient the diagnosis. Chronic obstructive pulmonary diseases show intense pulses and sweat. These patients receive iodinated expectorants and this can lead to the formation of a goiter, which obscures the condition. Exclusion of the above situations is by laboratory investigation.

a.vi. Treatment

Treatment of hyperthyroidism can be done with: 1. medicines; 2. radioactive iodine disruption; and 3. surgical intervention. Each treatment method has indications and contraindications and the choice of appropriate treatment is tailored to the circumstances. The rules of treatment are:

1. People under 40 years of age are treated with anti-thyroid drugs or with surgery. Treatment is started with medication unless there are particular reasons for preference for surgery. Treatment lasts for a long period of 1.5-2 years and for some for many years. If antihypertensive drugs fail or side effects occur, we resort to surgery. If a relapse occurs because of early discontinuation or incomplete treatment, treatment is repeated at the normal doses.

Surgery is preferred when the goiter is enormous or when due to the condition or personality of the patient, it is anticipated that long-term treatment and monitoring required when using drugs is difficult or impossible.

The administration of radioactive iodine is limited to cases of drug failure and relapse after surgery or when there is a failure to perform a surgical procedure. At very young ages (<20 years), radioactive iodine is given when inevitable. At the older age and as we approach the 40th year, the decision to use the radio-ion is taken with less hesitation.

2. After the age of 40, treatment begins with drugs, but radioactive iodine is more easily used when medication fails. In large and nodular goiters, surgery is recommended when the general condition of the patient is good.

- Pharmaceutical treatment. The pharmaceutical treatment of hyperthyroidism is aimed at reducing the production of thyroid hormones and treating their biological activity. For the inhibition of secretion of thyroid hormones, pyrimidine derivatives, propylthiouracil and imidazole derivatives or carbimazole and its methimazole derivative are used. The action of these antithyroid drugs is based on their inhibitory effect on the incorporation of iodine into the tyrosine molecule, the production of iodotyrosins (MIT and DIT) and their association to the formation of thyroid hormones. Propylthiouracil (PPT) has been found to have a peripheral effect because it inhibits the conversion of T4 to T3, more pronounced than imidazoles. In addition PPT passes harder than the placenta and the breast and is preferred in the treatment of hyperthyroidism during pregnancy. Carbimazole is given at the start of treatment at 30 mg daily in 3 doses. PPT is given every 6 hours at doses of 100-150 mg. This dose causes a decrease in thyroid hormone production to levels that are sometimes lower than normal. After the first or second month of treatment and if improvement has been achieved, the dose progressively decreases. For the risk of relapse, administration continues at maintenance doses over a long period of time even if complete withdrawal of symptoms occurs from the first months of treatment.

Anti-thyroid drugs may have mild and severe side effects. The slight side effects are hypersensitivity reactions such as rashes, pruritus, dermatitis or less fever, arthralgia, gastrointestinal disturbances. The annoyances are ruled out with the use of antihistamines and rarely need to stop treatment. The most serious side effect is blood and is agranulocytosis, which occurs more rarely, usually in the first weeks of treatment, without excluding its late onset. Patients are warned of the possibility of this side effect and given instructions for early recognition of first symptoms such as fever, sore throat, inflammation.

As an adjunct to the treatment of hyperthyroidism, drugs that inhibit β-adrenergic receptors and preferably propranolol are administered. Propranolol at doses ranging from 40-120 mg daily results in a rapid improvement in adrenergic manifestations (tachycardia, tremor, sweating) much faster than anti-thyroid medications and so the patient is totally or largely relieved of these symptoms until a decrease occurs of thyroid secretion by anti-thyroid therapy. When administering propanol, consideration should be given to the negative inotropic effect of the drug on the heart and its effect on myocardial conduction as well as the fact that, unlike anti-thyroid drugs, thyroid hormone synthesis and therefore its hyper-secretion does not influenced by the drug.

The advantages of the drug therapy are: a) that it is bloodless; b) it is effective in excess of 60%; c) the tolerance of medication by the patients is relatively good. The disadvantages of anti-thyroid medicines are: a) the need for long-term treatment, b) the appearance of side effects, c) the frequency of relapses.

- Radioactive iodine treatment. Treatment with radioactive iodine is based on the ability of thyroid to selectively retain iodine. Radioisotope is concentrated in the gland at high density and, due to its low radiation penetration, almost exclusively radiates thyroid tissue. In this way partial destruction of the gland is achieved which is capable of eliminating hyperthyroidism and at the same time avoids the damage of surrounding tissues. As radioisotope 131I is used, which emits 90% rays of β which have a penetration of a few millimeters in the thyroid tissue and 10% non-absorbed gamma rays. 131I has a half-life of 8 days. The use of 125I, which has a slower half-life, has not produced better results and has not worked out. The dose administered depends on the size of the goiter, the radioiodin retention rate and the severity of the condition. Doses of 10-15 mCi are usually administered.

Improvement of hyperthyroidism begins from the first month after treatment and is evident within three months. If no improvement is noted during this interval, a second dose is given. A smaller percentage of patients need more doses. After administration of the radioisotope and if the condition is severe or there is a need for immediate relief of the patient from certain symptoms (tachycardia e.t.c.), antihtyroid drugs or propranolol or both at the discretion of the physician and until the radioiodin acts.

The advantages of radioactive iodine therapy are: a) the risk of the method; b) its great simplicity; (simple ingestion of water containing radioisotope); c) the small financial burden on the patient; d) satisfactory efficiency

The drawbacks are two: a) the frequent induction of hypothyroidism, b) the possible radiation dangers.

The occurrence of hypothyroidism is common after radioactive iodine treatment, so regular monitoring of patients for many years is required to detect thyroid deficiency and early treatment with substitution to prevent its effects. The establishment of hypothyroidism is often slow and progressive and the symptoms are not interpreted correctly by the patient or attributed to other causes. The informed doctor, however, must detect and evaluate the first manifestations of the disease in patients who have received radioiodine to put the diagnosis as early as possible. The measurement of thyroid hormones in the blood (T4 and T3) and in particular the measurement of TSH, which is a sensitive indicator of thyroid dysfunction, helps diagnose. The potential risks of using radioactive iodine were thyroid cancer, leukemia, reproductive system damage and genetic damage.

- Surgery. Surgical treatment consists in removing a large part of the gland to eliminate the source of overproduction of thyroid hormones. The effectiveness of surgical treatment depends on the patient's good preparation and the surgeon's experience. Preparation is to reduce the symptoms of the disease by administering anti-thyroid drugs and propanol. The use of propanol alone is not recommended by most authors because the drug does not reduce the production of thyroid hormones, which is desirable to avoid the risk of thyrotoxic crisis during surgery. Some are also administered iodine in the form of potassium iodide preoperatively to improve the vascularity of the gland.

Surgical treatment has the advantages of: a) rapid relief from the disease, b) greater efficacy compared to the pharmaceutical treatment, c) removable nodules of goiter, d) when the goiter is large, the aesthetic effect is satisfactory due to the reduction of throat swelling.

The drawbacks are: a) post-operative complications; b) post-operative hypothyroidism; and c) the unsightly effect of scarring. Post-operative complications include bleeding, thyrotoxic crisis, hypoparathyroidism, and laryngeal nerve fever. Mortality during surgery in special centers is insignificant. The thyroid crisis is rare when the patient is well prepared. Hypoparathyroidism may be transient and permanent. Transient is quite common in thyroid surgery. Appears in the first few days after surgery and leaves after weeks or months. The permanent appears later and requires systematic treatment. Lower laryngeal nerve damage is a serious complication of the operation because it causes permanent disturbances of the voice. Postoperative hypothyroidism is not uncommon and usually occurs within the first two years of surgery.

b) Autonomous toxic adenoma

Hyperthyroidism can be caused by the hyper-secretion of thyroid hormones originating from adenoma (or rare adenomas) of the autonomic gland. The attributes of the adenoma are that it produces and secretes thyroid hormones without obeying stimulation or inhibitory stimuli. The autonomic toxic adenoma is also referred to as Plummer's disease. Plummer in 1913 described the existence of hyperthyroidism in people with goiter nodules and not only in people with diffuse goiter. For this Plummer's disease, most characterize hyperthyroidism with nodular goiter. On the contrary, the autonomous single toxic adenoma identified in 1947 when radioactive iodine was first used may be considered a separate form of hyperthyroidism. The frequency of the toxic adenoma varies, but it is estimated to be 10-15% of all cases of hyperthyroidism. The adenoma is more common in women (8: 1) and in adults over 45 years of age.

b.i. Rationale

Two types of mutations have been observed in a significant percentage of toxic adenomas, one involving a mutation of the Gs protein, which converts it into the gsp oncogene which induces intense stimulation of adenylyl cyclase and the second relates to a TSH receptor site mutation localized to the amino acids of the inter-membrane region. Both mutations result in autonomous and intense hyper-function of the thyroid cell.

b.ii. Pathological Physiology

The autonomic adenoma produces thyroxine and T3 in amounts that can cause symptoms of hyperthyroidism. The sensitivity of tissue to TSH is no greater than normal thyroid, and yet hormone synthesis occurs at a faster and more intense pace. Iodine intake, thyroid hormone formation and thyroglobulin are elevated. When autonomic production of thyroid hormones from the adenoma reaches large amounts, TSH secretion is inhibited, resulting in sub-function of the remaining thyroid parenchyma, except for the adenoma.

b.iii. Symptomology

Growth of the adenoma may be slow and may take years to become clinically perceptible or symptomatic. The production of thyroid hormones from the adenoma may be moderate in amount or only slightly elevated and maintained at this level for a long time without apparent symptomatology. For these reasons, the symptoms caused by the autonomic adenoma are generally milder and lighter and therefore their clinical finding is more difficult. From the eyes there is only the contraction of the eyelids and never prolapse or edema of the eyelids. Thyroid adenoma always grope in the form of nodules, since to give symptoms must acquire dimensions over 2cm. The nodule is circumscribed, grows slowly and has a semi-hard texture. Characteristic of the autonomic adenoma is that the remaining thyroid is normal or degraded. Thyroid nodule is usually the only cause of patients coming to the doctor. Tachycardia is less intense but sometimes, on vulnerable soil, complete arrhythmia or heart failure is observed. Terror, weight loss and muscle weakness are less pronounced in the toxic adenoma. The thermophobia may not be perceived by the patients and is detected in hot hands and fine sweating. Nervousness manifests itself with vague and not characteristic symptoms. Hyperthyroidism with its complete symptomatology is observed in about 25% of patients.

b.iv. Laboratory findings

The lack of a clear clinical picture in the toxic adenoma is compensated by pathognomonic laboratory findings. The most characteristic is the scintigraphic image of the thyroid in which, instead of the contour of the entire gland, only a round oval area, called hot nodule is deleted. TSH administration confirms the diagnosis when the blood hormones are normal and there is a suspicion that there is a single lobe, or the lobe that is not depicted is destroyed and therefore is not deleted. In the toxic adenoma TSH induces stimulation of the healthy thyroid parenchyma that was in a functional inactivity due to inhibition of endogenous TSH and thus in the scintigraphy the whole gland is deleted.

In some cases, the adenoma is seen in the scan as an area that retains the radioiodin at a higher concentration than the rest of the thyroid, which shows a weak or just deleted retention. In this case, which is characterized as scintigraphic lukewarm nodule, it adenoma which produces several hormones to completely inhibit TSH and thus the thyroid shows rudimentary functionality. Clinically, the tepid nodules do not give symptoms other than local swelling of the thyroid, but need to be monitored because it can migrate after unknown time in toxic adenomas.

Thyroid hormones are elevated or at higher normal levels and TSH characteristics are suppressed in the toxic adenoma. During the development of an adenoma, which may last for years, it is not uncommon to find normal thyroid hormone levels in the blood. TRH stimulation showing a lack of TSH response showing a lack of TSH response reveals the abnormality earlier than the increase in thyroid hormone.

b.v. Treatment

Treatment of the toxic adenoma is preferably surgical. In cases where surgery is impossible, therapeutic radioactive iodine is administered in large doses, or anti-thyroid drugs.

c. Polycystic toxic goitre

The polycystic toxic goiter comes from a long-gone goiter and has undergone morphological changes that result in functional autonomy, which is intense, manifests itself as hyperthyroidism. The overactive parts of the thyroid parenchyma is usually accumulation hull in nodules and follicles. Their origins from a pre-existing goiter mean that up to the stage of hyperactivity and hypersecretion, two stages of varying duration are mediated: a single goiter stage and a transition stage with clinical hyperthyroidism.

The formation of the nodes is a result of a combination and cooperative action of genes or growth stimulants and inhibition of inhibitory or growth factor activity. Polycystic goiter is mainly seen in the elderly because it is usually necessary for many years for simple goiter to become toxic. The diagnosis is triggered by high T4 and T3 values and low TSH. A diagnostic and therapeutic problem exists when the values are marginal or when the T4 and T3 values are normal, but there is suppressed TSH, which does not react to TRH. The diagnostic problem in these cases, which can be described as subclinical or potential hyperthyroidism, is also associated with the treatment to be applied in these cases. The decision will depend on the age, size and texture of the goiter, the general condition, the cardiovascular function and the evolution of the condition. In the case of clinical hyperthyroidism the treatment is with anti-thyroid drugs or surgery and possibly radioactive iodine.

d. Hyperthyroidism in acute thyroiditis

Acute thyroiditis during the initial phase of inflammatory processes shows increased release of thyroid hormones and symptoms of hyperthyroidism. The duration of this phase varies, and the hyperthyroid events are covered by other symptoms of inflammation that are intense in most cases of acute thyroiditis (tachycardia, fever, anxiety, etc.). In some forms of acute thyroiditis the clinical manifestations of inflammation are mild and thus the symptoms of hyperthyroidism predominate and may lead to classic long-term treatment in a form of the disease that is transient. Treatment of hyperthyroidism during acute thyroiditis should be discontinued to ascertain whether the gland function has returned to normal.

e. Specific forms of hyperthyroidism

T3 Hyperthyroidism

The ability to measure T4 and T3 separately in the blood of patients with thyroid disorders revealed the presence of hyperthyroidism in which blood T4 is normal but T3 is elevated. Many times, this situation is a preliminary stage after which it increases and T4, but sometimes remains permanently high only the T3. The clinical picture does not from the case where both thyroid hormones are elevated. The incidence of T3 hyperthyroidism is not great, but the knowledge of the existence of this form of disease protects us from the mistake of rejecting the diagnosis in individuals with obvious clinical symptoms in which T4 was found normal without T3 being measured at the same time. T3 hyperthyroidism is most commonly seen in the elderly and relapse of the disease, particularly after surgery or radioiodine therapy.

T4 Hyperthyroidism

Cases of hyperthyroidism with increased T4 and normal T3 have been reported. These cases were observed in patients who had concomitant hyperthyroidism with some other severe disease. Also in patients who experienced hyperthyroidism after iodine administration. The hyperthyroidal condition in the latter cases was transient.

f. Hyperthyroidism and pregnancy

Hyperthyroidism may occur during pregnancy in a patient suffering from hyperthyroidism. The problem of the disease and the treatment applied to the progression of pregnancy and the fetus is raised. The fertility of women with mild or moderate hyperthyroidism is usually not affected and pregnancy is possible. Pregnancy may also occur in a woman in whom hyperthyroidism is under the control of anti-thyroid medicines. Diagnosis of hyperthyroidism during pregnancy presents difficulties, because pregnant women show due to pregnancy certain manifestations of hyperthyroidism, such as tachycardia, thermophobia, low thyroid swelling. Premenopausal pregnancy has a frequent occurrence of hyperthyroidism during pregnancy. Any weight loss is covered by weight gain during pregnancy. The increase in T4 (TBG)-globin, observed in pregnancy by estrogen, causes an increase in total T4 of the blood. For this in pregnancy, it is best to take into account the value of free T4 and T3 and the index of free thyroxine for the diagnosis of hyperthyroidism or the finding of euthyroid status. Treatment of hyperthyroidism during pregnancy is done with antithyroid drugs or with surgery. The use of radioactive iodine is contraindicated. Iodine should also not be used therapeutically in pregnancy because it passes through the placenta and causes inhibition of fetal thyroid hormone production resulting in large goiter or hypothyroidism. The anti-thyroid drugs passes through the placenta and is therefore administered in small, relatively, doses to improve hyperthyroidism. With this tactic, drug therapy controls hyperthyroidism without adverse effects on the fetus, despite the theoretical risks. Thyroid hormones, however, have difficulty passing the placenta so that the fetus is dependent on hormones derived from the function of its own thyroid. Surgery, if considered necessary, occurs in the second trimester of pregnancy after a pharmaceutical preparation. Childbirth in pregnant women with hyperthyroidism is not particularly troublesome, but obstetricians should be aware of the possibility of hyperthyroidism in neonates. Chronic thyroiditis, which is rarely postpartum, can be manifested by an increase in thyroid hormones and hyperthyroid symptoms. The condition characterized as postpartum hyperthyroidism is transient or may turn into hypothyroidism.

g. Neonatal hyperthyroidism

Hyperthyroidism in neonates is a serious condition observed in newborns that their mothers showed in the pregnancy of hyperthyroidism, free or untreated. The disease, due to the maternal thyroid immunoglobulus passage in the fetus, is rare, but its mortality, if not diagnosed in time, is great. Hyperthyroidism usually manifests itself from the first few hours after delivery and is characterized by extraophthalmia, goiter, tachycardia, sweating, body-twitching and hyperactivity, continuous crying. Tachycardia is sometimes significant and is accompanied by signs of heart failure (hepatomegaly, cyanosis). Gastrointestinal symptoms, such as diarrhea and vomiting, may disorient the diagnosis. High thyroid hormone levels are found in the blood of the newborns. The diagnosis, when maternal hyperthyroidism is known, is not difficult. The treatment consists of the administration of anti-thyroid drugs and beta-blockers and the symptomatic treatment of various events. If the first critical days pass, the symptoms go away within 2-3 months, except for the extra-longest one. The urgency of neonatal hyperthyroidism is due to the fact that maternal antibodies are metabolized and disappear. In the case of neonatal hyperthyroidism with complete and intense symptomatology, which is rare, there should be much more in which the disease manifests itself in a lighter form that escapes diagnosis. The presence of high TSH-RAb titers in the mother favors the emergence of neonatal hyperthyroidism.

h. Childhood hyperthyroidism

The onset of hyperthyroidism during childhood creates diagnostic and therapeutic problems due to the non-classical manifestation of the disease, its impact on child growth and the difficulty of treatment. The frequency of hyperthyroidism in children, although much lower than hypothyroidism, is not insignificant. It is estimated that 7% of all cases of hyperthyroidism, involving children under 15, but among thyroid diseases in childhood, the disease is 10%. More than half of the patients are more than 10 years old. The superiority of females is maintained and is great: 3-6 females to 1 male.

h.i. Rationale

It is noteworthy that the greatest number of cases of hyperthyroidism in children shows a diffuse toxic adenoma. The toxic adenoma is rare. Etiology is attributed to the presence of thyroid-inducing immunoglobulins. The aggravating factors for the onset of the disease are: a) the presence of thyroid abnormality (simple goiter, hyper or hypothyroidism) in parents or the family; b) emotional disturbances due to intra-familial friction.

h.ii. Symptomology

All symptoms of the disease may be present in children, but the symptomatology is dominated by two phenomena: a) behavioral and character disorder due to the psychiatric manifestations of the disease; and b) the effects on physical growth. Symptoms may appear abruptly or gradually, so the diagnosis is difficult and delayed.

Behavioral disorders are the reason why parents usually seek help from the doctor. Great emotion, irritability, neurotic manifestations, easy anger and crying and generally psycho-social instability and inability to concentrate, create problems in family and school. Changes in the rate of body growth are common and characteristic in children's hyperthyroidism. There is an acceleration of body growth, which may precede the onset of other symptoms or dominate the clinical picture. It is usually accompanied by reduced body weight despite good or increased appetite. Weight reduction is less important than in adults and due to polyphagia, weight loss is sometimes absent or even observed. At the same time as the acceleration of body growth, a faster maturation of the skeleton occurs, resulting in bone age being greater than the chronological one. The other symptoms are in varying proportions and intensity. The exophthalmos is usually in the form of retraction of the upper eyelid or glowing look. The goiter is small, always diffuse and homogeneous in the composition. Tachycardia is evident and usually exceeds 120 stiffness. It increases in the thrills for this to be checked at home by parents in a resting state of the patient or during sleep. Endurance is not a solid finding. However, hyperactivity is often continuous and unnecessary that can take the form of chorionic movements. Thermophobia and muscle weakness can be observed in a large number of cases.

h.iii. Laboratory finding and diagnosis

Laboratory findings are the same as in adults and allow diagnosis in doubtful cases. The differential diagnosis will be made by the simple goiter and efsiglinita people with neurotic manifestations.

h.iv. Treatment

Treatment of hyperthyroidism in children is done with anti-thyroid medicines or with surgery. Anti-thyroid medications are used as in adults with dose adjustment according to the age and weight of the patient. Treatment continues for a long time. Relapses are common and are due largely to incomplete treatment due to patient disrespect or lack of family unity and co-operation. Surgical treatment is applied if drug therapy fails or in case of relapses or when conditions do not allow for long-term treatment with drugs. Very rarely and only in exceptional cases where no other treatment can be administered, hence delivers therapeutically radioactive iodine.

i.Senile Hyperthyroidism

Hyperthyroidism in people over 60 years of age is not uncommon but remains often undiagnosed for three reasons: a) why the frequency of its existence is neglected; b) why one of the two main symptoms of the disease, the ectopic and the goiter, are absent or not evident in 2/3 of the cases and c) why the manifestation of hyperthyroidism are attributable to other conditions.

The incidence of disease in people over 60 years ranges between 10-17% of all patients. The female to male relationship is 4: 1.

Many cases of senile hyperthyroidism are due to nodular toxic goiter or toxic adenoma. In the first case, it is old gooes that developed nodules that functioned autonomously.

Among the elicitors, mental trauma is common. Extreme illnesses, like flu, are sometimes the principle of installing hyperthyroidism.

Taking iodinated drugs, such as amiodarone, can be the cause of hyperthyroidism in this case.

Symptoms are established slowly and asynchronously, in a way that the disease is manifested for a long time. Early or no diagnosis depends on the presence of at least one of the two classic symptoms that automatically drives thinking into hyperthyroidism: the ectopic and the goiter. Ectoplasty exists in 50-64% of patients and in most cases is in low eyelid contractility. The goiter is found in 2/3 of the patients and is usually moderate in volume. Tachycardia is one of the most common symptoms. It is accompanied by a high rate of extraordinary contractions or complete arrhythmia or heart failure. Weight loss is also characteristic and intense in the elderly hyperthyroid. The frequency and intensity of other symptoms varies. When there is a loss of weight in the elderly without a certain cause, as well as frequent extraordinary contractions or heart failure, the possibility of hyperthyroidism, which is easily detected in laboratory, may be investigated. Some cases of hyperthyroidism in the elderly and without classic ectopic have been called "abnormal hyperthyroidism" or "covered hyperthyroidism".

In the treatment of hyperthyroidism in the elderly, radioactive iodine with which the disease is cured and a greater improvement in the condition is preferred. Particularly beneficial is the therapeutic effect on heart function, since complete arrhythmia and heart failure are attributed to 50% of the cases.

j. Thyroid edema crisis

The thyroid edema crisis is an exacerbation of the symptoms of hyperthyroidism to an extent that endangers the patient's life. In the past, the classical form of the thyroid crisis occurred during surgery to treat hyperthyroidism in patients with pre-operative treatment insufficient. In addition to surgery, other stressful conditions such as infections, injuries, surgery, intense emotional factors are the cause of the crisis. Sudden discontinuation of drug therapy or, more rarely, therapeutic administration of radioactive iodine can cause the crisis. The exacerbation of the symptoms occurs abruptly and rapidly after the excretory cause. Patients have great anxiety and agitation and persistent hyperactivity. At the same time hyperpyrexia, peripheral vasodilation and hot saddle skin are observed throughout the body. Tachycardia is large, usually more than 150 beats and can lead to heart failure and pulmonary edema. Diarrhea and vomiting are common like swelling of the liver and light jaundice. Still there are manic manifestations and mental confusion, the patient falls into coma and most of the time ends up if the appropriate therapeutic measures are not taken. The mortality rate of the crisis is high if the appropriate measures are not taken.

The pathogenesis of the thyrotoxic crisis has not been fully elucidated. It is believed to be due to the release of large amounts of thyroid hormones in the circulation. However, the level of thyroid hormones in the blood during the crisis is not particularly high.

The diagnosis of the crisis in its classical event is not difficult. This is a hyperthyroid patient who, after a stressful strain, suddenly shows a great outburst of his symptoms.

Treatment of a mild type of thyroid dystocia is symptomatic and not difficult. But addressing the severe crisis requires active two-way measures to be taken: (a) to reduce the production of thyroid hormones; and (b) to combat dangerous clinical manifestations. To deal with the hyper-secretion of thyroid hormones, anti-thyroid drugs are administered at high doses by the oral or gastric tube. Carbimazole is given at the 20 mg dose and the propylthiouracil at the 300 mg dose every 3-6 hours. The latter is preferred because of its peripheral effect on T3 inhibition by T4. Iodine in the form of Lugol if used to inhibit secretion of thyroid hormones should always be given after anti-thyroid medications to be administered after anti-thyroid drugs to not serve as a raw material for thyroid hormone synthesis. Symptomatic treatment includes the administration of: a) β-receptor blockers to inhibit adrenergic events such as tachycardia, sweating, tremor, etc. Propanol is administered at a dose of 20-80 mg orally every 4-6 hours and / 2 mg intravenously. In the event of heart failure, cardiotonics are administered. (b) Whey protein to which cortisone is added (150-300 mg daily). Serum needs range between 2500-4000 ml per day depending on dehydration. (c) Barbiturates and reserpins for inhibition of the central nervous system. At the same time hyperpyrexia is treated with the use of ice patches. In spite of intensive treatment, the mortality of the serious form of the thyroid dystocia crisis remains severe. For this reason, the best treatment is considered to be its intake by applying all the necessary measures, so that the treatment of hyperthyroidism is normal and seamless.

k. Thyroid ophthalmopathy

The ophthalmological manifestations of hyperthyroidism are due to the effect of thyroid hormones on immune factors, including contraction of the eyelids, infiltration and muscle weakness of ocular muscles, retinal tissue infiltration and eyelid edema. Thyroid hormones cause the contraction of the eyelids with an adrenergic mechanism that is removed by administering β-blockers. Increasing the retrobulbar tissue, causing the prolapse of the bulb, infiltration of eye muscles and edema of the eyelids does not come from an increase of thyroid hormone blood. The pathogenesis of these lesions is not fully elucidated, but the immune mechanism of the lesions is believed to be certain. The lesion originates from anti-thyroid immunoglobulins produced by lymphocytes following thyroid antigen or antigens produced by the fibroblasts or other cells. Pathological lesions consist of infiltration of connective tissue by lymphocytes and plasmocytes, an increase in fibroblasts and the accumulation of glycosaminoglycans. Muscles are similarly infiltrated and increased in volume and degeneration. Ejaculation of this form may follow independent progression from the course of hyperthyroidism.

Two extreme forms of thyroid ophthalmopathy are: a) Euthyroidal ophthalmopathy; and b) its severe form of endangering vision.

Euthyroidal ophthalmopathy is called ophthalmopathy which is not accompanied by any clinical point of hyperthyroidism. Thyroid hormones in the blood are normal. In many patients, TRH does not induce TSH stimulation or T3 administration does not inhibit radioiodine retention or anti-thyroid antibodies in the blood, as occurs in hyperthyroidism. The condition may remain stagnant for many years or switch to clinical hyperthyroidism or experience a slow improvement.

The severe and dangerous form of thyroid ophthalmopathy is characterized by a large, progressive and asymmetric prolapse of bulbs, significant eyelid swelling, ocular paralysis, conjunctivitis, corneal lesions and visual disturbances that may result in blindness. Ophthalmologic lesions in this form appear progressively, usually in patients during the treatment of hyperthyroidism and are independent of the outcome of the treatment. The dangers to vision are great in this form of bruising, which is seen in approximately 5% of patients.

The treatment of bruising is difficult and its results unsatisfactory. The main treatment of excreta is with cortisone formulations which are administered in large doses for a sufficient period of time. Thyroid hormones are also provided for the patient to be fully euthyroid. At the same time protective measures are taken of the eyes with collires or in need of blepharophobia, for the protection of the cornea or even with relieving pruritus. Routine radiotherapy is recommended to inhibit the progressive development of bruising and / or prophylactic treatment.

1. Local myxedema

In some hyperthyroidal patients, localized myxedematic skin lesions, called local myxedema, appear. The lesions are related to the anterior and lateral surface of the lower part of the tibia and are therefore called prominent myxedema. They appear in the form of plaques, single or fuzzy, that have a complexion of blue and are usually large and symmetrical in both shins. Histologically, skin mucopolysaccharide infiltration of the skin has been identified, such as myxedema. The adjacent skin is normal. Local myxedema often accompanies the severe form of thyroid ophthalmopathy and occurs in less than 5% in hyperthyroid patients. In most cases it automatically drops off. When persistent, topical cortisone preparations are administered.

8.3 Goiter

Any swelling of the thyroid is called the goiter. Swelling of the thyroid due to regressive glandular hyperplasia without being accompanied by hormone hyper-secretion is called simple or non-toxic goiter. Increase in thyroid volume caused by neoplasms or inflammation of the gland is not classified in the simple goiter. Simple goiters are divided into endemic or sporadic. Endemic is called the goiter when it affects a large proportion of the population (> 10%), while the occurrence of individual cases in a country or place is characterized as sporadic goiter. The difference is quantitative. The simple goiter is distinguished in diffuse and nodular, depending on its morphological or histological characteristics. These are not different forms but evolutionary stages of the same disease. Simple goiter is considered to be the most widespread endocrinopathy in the world. The frequency in the female sex is 7-9 times higher than that of men. Simple goiter in most cases does not cause significant damage to the health of the sufferers. However, in some cases where the abnormality is severe, the malfunction of the thyroid has severe effects on the body. In all patients, there is a possibility that the simple goiter may grow into tumor and become nodular, creating both a sensory problem and a diagnostic dilemma on the existence of neoplasia, which requires special investigation.

a. **Rationale**

The main cause of the simple goiter, especially for the endemic appearance, is the inadequate iodine intake with food, due to inadequate soil content in iodine. However, the effect of other factors is also necessary. The higher incidence of goiter in women than in men, in certain families and in puberty, implies the presence of hereditary or predisposing factors favoring the appearance of the simple goiter. Local dietary habits, such as inadequate protein intake or eating of bronchial substances, may contribute to the development of the goiter. Various periods of female life in which there are increased thyroid hormone needs or hormonal upset, such as pregnancy, puberty, menopause, are bleeding factors when there is predisposition. Certain drugs that inhibit the function of thyroid enzymes have bronchoconstrictor activity. Iodine can also cause large amounts of goblet because it inhibits the binding of iodine to tyrosine.

b. Dystrophic goiters

Hormoneogenesis disorders due to congenital or hereditary disorders of thyroid enzymes responsible for the synthesis of thyroid hormones or pathological thyroglobulin may be the operative factors of the simple goiter. Damage, regardless of where it is seated, involves a reduced production of thyroid hormones, which leads to the formation of a goiter. When an abnormality of hormoneogenesis is important, it occurs apart from the goiter and hypothyroidism.

The frequency of hormone abnormalities that are related and inherited by the residual character has not been ascertained why many cases remain undiagnosed.

The classification of the anomalies in 5 categories:

- Thyroid iodine anomaly abnormal. The rare condition in which the thyroid fails to retain iodine. Salivary glands and gastric mucosa exhibit the same anomaly. The thyroid contains minimal iodine and is hyperplastic. Upon administration of radioactive iodine, 90% of the dose is excreted in the urine.
- Abnormal binding of iodine to tyrosine. It is the most common form of thyroid hormone disorder. Due to lack or insufficiency of peroxidase. Iodine fixation is high, but iodine retained can easily be pushed out of the gland by potassium perchlorate because it is not linked to an organic compound. This is the basis for a diagnostic test in which, after taking a diagnostic dose of radioactive iodine, potassium perchlorate is administered, in which case a sudden decrease in thyroid radioactivity due to radioiodine discharging remained unresponsive. This abnormality is seen in conjunction with congenital deafness and is called Pendred's syndrome.
- Tyrosine conjugation anomaly to produce thyroid hormones. It is only detected by thyroid tissue analysis, which contains large amounts of MIT and DIT and minimal T4 and T3, and therefore the actual incidence of the disorder is unknown.
- Anaphylaxis of iodotyrosins. Upon release of T4 and T3 from thyroglobulin, iodothyrosines are simultaneously replicated by a deiodinase to reuse iodine from the thyroid. Anomalies in the action of this enzyme result in the passage of significant amounts of MIT and DIT into the circulation, which did not crumble, excretion with urine and loss of iodine from the body and the formation of a goiter. The administration of radioactive MIT by mouth and its detection in unchanged form in urine demonstrates deficiency of deiodinase activity.

- Production of pathological thyroglobulin with different physicochemical properties than normal.

It became apparent that the center of the abnormalities was thyroglobulin, which had a pathological texture and properties resulting from its biosynthetic disorders. The abnormality of thyroglobulin may involve disorders: a. Genes regulating thyroglobulin biosynthesis; b. Transferring thyroglobulin from its locus of production to the thyroid gland, c. The addition of carbohydrate groups to its molecule, d. Its iodination, e. Its degradation. These abnormalities have an impact on the production and release of thyroid hormones. They also have consequences and in other phases of hormoneogenesis, which are not normal when there is pathological thyroglobulin. On the other hand, the presence of a normal amount of iodine in the thyroid is necessary to maintain the normal tertiary form of the thyroglobulin molecule and the iodine deficiency in turn causes additional anomalies in the thyroglobulin structure.

c. Pathological physiology

The creation of the simple goiter is done with the same mechanism regardless of the causative cause. The primary cause of excretion is the reduced production of thyroid hormones, which is a stimulant stimulus for the secretion of thyroid stimulating hormone according to the principle of regurgitation. TSH secreted stimulates thyroid hormone synthesis but also causes gland hyperplasia. Hormone synthesis, however, despite the stimulation is not normal due to the initial anomaly responsible for the reduced production of thyroid hormones and therefore does not result in the secretion of satisfactory amounts of hormones. As a result of this situation there are two possibilities: a) Thyroid secretion remains permanently hypo-physiological, and the mechanism of TSH regurgitation continues, causing large gland hyperplasia. b) Due to TSH, the gland manages to produce hormonal amounts sufficient for the body's needs and enough to stop the stimulation of TSH secretion. However, once TSH overproduction ceases, the initial state of reduced thyroid hormone production is restored, causing a new TSH secretory wave and a new thyroid hyperplasia phase. In the first case the swelling of the gland is progressive and the goiter has large dimensions. In the second case, the increase in gland volume is performed by reductions corresponding to each period of hyper-secretion of TSH. In both cases, hyperplasia is counterbalanced and aims at increasing the hormone secretion mass by increasing the number of cells to compensate for the fact that the hormone production capacity of each cell constituting the secretory unit is reduced. Thyroid hyperplasia in the simple goiter does not result in hyper-secretion of thyroid hormones for the simplest reason that as soon as secretion reaches the normal limits, further stimulation of TSH secretion is automatically interrupted. Hyperplasia is initially accompanied by hypertrophy of thyroid cells, which show signs of intense functional activity.

Thyroid vesicles exhibit a small lumen, fold wall and cubic or cylindrical cells. Over time the epithelium is delaminated and shows evidence of functional inertia, the lumen grows and fills with colloid. This image of subversion may be adjacent to regions with intense functionality. These morphological alterations are due to the functional phases of calmness and super-function that succeed one another. Effect of continuous functional and morphological gland disorder is bladder formation, adenoma development, cystic hemorrhage with scarring or deposition of calcium salts, inflammatory reactions and histological morphology of long-term bronchial glands and their nodular appearance. The concentration of iodine in the thyroid by gram of tissue is reduced to the simple goiter. It is usually 100 μg / g versus normal 500 μg / g. In addition, a section of iodine trapped in regions of the gland that do not exhibit normal functionality and thus does not participate in hormone synthesis. Therefore, although iodine may be normal due to the large volume of the gland, there is endotriotic iodine deficiency. The amount of thyroglobulin is also decreased in the goiter. The content of T4 and DIT is clearly reduced and the amount of MIT it contains is increased. This results in an increase in the MIT / DIT ratio and the production of more T3 and less T4 than normal individuals. Blood TSH is usually normal in the simple goiter, except for cases where blood levels of T4 and T3 are low. The increase in TSH occurs in the early stages of the disease and the subsequent continuation of the pathophysiological mechanism requires shorter or shorter exactions of TSH secretion. There is also evidence that TSH activity in the thyroid is stronger when there is local iodine deficiency. Thyroid hormones in the blood are normal or at the lower normal range. Analogically, there is a tendency to lower T4 and less T3.

d. Symptomology

In most cases the increase in thyroid volume is slow and progressive and does not cause discomfort to the patient except local swelling. The goiter can get large dimensions without causing symptoms. In rare cases, the swelling of the gland causes convincing phenomena resulting in dysparesis and more rarely dysphonia. Local swelling is usually evident with the review. The palpation will reveal the composition of the gland and its limits. In the large goiter, cervix and chest pain are observed by vascular pressure. Expansion of the goiter to the anterior medulla can degrade the trachea. The surface of the gland is smooth or shows abnormalities in the form of the warts. The constellation of the gland in the recent bronchi is homogeneous and soft over the palpable area. In drones that are long-lasting or those that have developed abruptly, the composition is usually elastic, semi-hard and nodular.

e. Diagnosis

Diagnosis of the goiter is easy and can be done with a clinical examination. With the review, the anterior cervical surface is swollen. Swelling becomes sometimes more apparent when swallowed, followed by movements of thyroid cartilage. The backward head is a handy way for young children to reveal the goiter. The palpation reveals the size of the gland and its composition. The exact thyroid and parenchymal boundaries are determined by ultrasound and scintigraphic functionality. The big problem of simple goiter is not the finding but its differential diagnosis from the three other conditions that present with thyroid swelling: hyperthyroidism, thyroiditis and thyroid cancer. The simple goiter is easily distinguishable from hyperthyroidism due to the absence of characteristic symptoms of gland over-activity and is confirmed by the measurement of thyroid hormones and TSH. Blocking or detecting symptoms allows for accurate diagnosis and protects the patient not only from unnecessary but also harmful treatment if a wrong diagnosis is made. Particularly harmful is the administration of anti-thyroids in the event that a simple bronchocellus is mistakenly perceived as hyperthyroidism, because swelling of the gland will be aggravated by inhibition of hormoneogenesis caused by anti-thyroid drugs. Thyroiditis will be diagnosed with more difficulty. Subacute thyroiditis from local pain, generic phenomena and the appearance of swelling at the same time with these events. Chronic thyroiditis by finding high titers of anti-thyroid antibodies in blood, gland composition and ultrasound image, which is often characteristic. Thyroid cancer presents more serious diagnostic problems. Recent diffuse swelling of the gland, which has a homogeneous and soft texture, does not pose a differential diagnosis problem with thyroid cancer. Conversely, the nodular goiter, in which one or more hard focuses in the form of a nodule or vagina are palpable, need to be separated from the cancer. The distinction is not easy. The harsh texture, uneven surface and shape, rapid growth, adhesion to surrounding tissues, large larynx, lymph angularity are in favor of cancer. However, the absence of these elements does not at all provide the certainty that it is a simple goiter that does not house a carcinoma. Recourse to ultrasound, scintigraphy and, in particular, fine needle biopsy is essential for differential diagnosis.

f. Treatment

The treatment of simple goiter is pharmaceutical or surgical. Conservative treatment consists of daily administration of thyroxine (100-200 μg L-T4) to inhibit TSH and suppress glandular hyperplasia. In this treatment, small, recent, and diffuse goiters respond well. Patients continue to be treated for a long time and repeat it if during the discontinuation the thyroid shows signs of swelling. Surgical treatment is applied to nodular goiters (especially when there is evidence of cancer or when there are large and many oocytes that are not functional in the scintigraphy or do not occupy much of the thyroid), large goiters (when they do not retreat with conservative therapy), when there are pressures and finally for aesthetic reasons.

8.4 Thyroiditis

In addition to the specific and purulent thyroid inflammations (eg tuberculosis, staphylococcal infection), which are extremely rare and have no effect other than local disaster, more frequently occurring inflammatory conditions of the gland causing transient hyper or under function. Permanent subfunction may also be a consequence of a thyroiditis. Thyroiditis of this kind can be distinguished in three forms:

a. Sub-acute thyroiditis or thyroiditis of De Quervain

Sub-acute thyroiditis affects women more often, especially among women aged 30-50 years, is rare in children, lasts from a few days to several months, is automatically killing without causing permanent thyroid injury, but is often recurrent. It rarely causes hypothyroidism possibly when there is chronic thyroiditis. The actual incidence of the disease is not easy to ascertain because it usually escapes diagnosis because it is perceived as a common soreness.

a.i. Rationale

Sub-acute thyroiditis is an acute inflammatory disease of the thyroid gland, probably due to a viral infection. Various viruses have been implicated, such as mumps virus, Coxsackie viruses and adenoviruses, either due to the detection of the virus in biopsy specimens taken from the gland or by the detection in blood of increased antibody titers against the virus during the infection.

a.ii. Pathological physiology

The inflammatory processes occupy the entire gland and are characterized by the infiltration of the vesicles by lymphocytes and giant cells, the colloid reduction, the hyperplasia of the wall cells and the increase in the size of the vesicles to rupture. Pathologic anomalies cause functional thyroid disorders: retention of iodine is low, thyroid hormone synthesis is reduced and stimulation with TSH is unresponsive. At the same time, the damaged vesicles are released in abundance by thyroglobulin and thyroid hormones and other iodinated substances. The sequence of events is usually the following: during the first phase thyroid function is suppressed but at the same time release of thyroid hormones and causing mild symptoms of hyperthyroidism, depending on the severity of the disease. In the second phase, the thyroid hormone stores are depleted, new hormones are difficult to produce because of the ongoing inflammatory reaction and consequently the occurrence of hypo-thyroidic events is likely. The third phase is characterized by automatic healing and restoration of gland function. Establishing permanent hypothyroidism is rare.

a.iii. Symptomology

The symptomatology of the disease is characterized by three clinical elements: a) local phenomena; b) general phenomena; and c) thyroid disorder. The clinical picture depends on the severity of the disease and its phase. In the first stage of the disease, there is a painful swelling of the gland. The pain is reflected in the lateral cervix, ears and jaws. Usually there is pain during swallowing. Swelling is small or moderate, tough and sometimes asymmetrical. The local effects of pain are accompanied by general phenomena such as fever, chills, headache, myalgia, malaise. The symptoms of hyperthyroidism present at this stage (tachycardia, thermophobia, light tremor) are difficult to distinguish between other symptoms of inflammation. A form of disease without local pain and with severe thyroid overactive symptoms can be diagnosed as hyperthyroidism. The effects of hyperthyroidism can lead to long-term anti-thyroid therapy while being transient. Thyroiditis is diagnosed by low radioiodine retention. In the second stage, which lasts longer than the first, the local symptoms remain in the form of sensitivity to the palpation of the thyroid, or as automatic alveolus or stiffness or simple swelling of the gland. General phenomena are unclear and take the form of fever, strength, generalized malaise and anorexia. At this stage, thyroid dysfunction may be generalized enough to manifest itself clinically.

a.iv. Laboratory findings

Laboratory findings vary according to the course of the disease. Initially, T4 and T3 are high, while TSH and thyroid uptake of radioactive iodine are particularly low. The sedimentation velocity of the reds is particularly high. Anti-thyroid antibodies are not usually detected in serum. As the disease progresses, T4 and T3 recede, TSH increases and symptoms of hypothyroidism appear. Later, the uptake of radioactive iodine increases, reflecting the recovery of the gland from the acute insult.

a.v. Diagnosis

Sub-acute thyroiditis can be distinguished from other viral diseases due to thyroid infestation. It is distinguished from Graves disease because it exhibits low intake of radioactive iodine with high T3 and T4 in the serum and suppressed TSH, while no anti-thyroid antibodies are detected.

a.vi. Treatment

Treatment of sub-acute thyroiditis is symptomatic. The main therapeutic agent is symptomatic. The main therapeutic agent is the administration of cortisone which results in immediate and spectacular results within 24 hours. Cortisone, though relieving symptoms, does not seem to change the course of the disease. Administration is done with high initial doses (20-40 mg of prednisone) maintained for several days and then progressively reduced. During interruption, the symptoms may reappear, so the treatment is repeated. Some administer concurrently with cortisone and thyroxine at substitution doses.

b. Lymphocytic thyroiditis or Hashimoto's disease

Chronic lymphocytic thyroiditis or Hashimito disease is the most common form of non-specific thyroiditis and the most common cause of hypothyroidism and is likely to be one of the most common thyroid diseases. Its incidence is estimated at 1-2% of the population based on serological or pathological examinations. It affects 9 times more often females, especially those aged 50-60 years.

b.i. Rationale

Hashimoto's thyroiditis is considered to be an autoimmune disease of the endocrine system. Patients' blood is mainly anti-thyroglobulin antibodies (TgAb), anti-peroxidase (TPOAb) and TSH receptor blocking antibodies [TSH-R (block)]. Antithyroglobulin antibodies are found in the largest number of patients with Hashimoto's thyroiditis and high title in the early stages of the disease and may later be reduced or disappear. There are also many patients with underlying and hyperthyroidism. Anti-thyroid antibodies against TPO-Ab peroxidase or microsomal antibodies are thyroid and human-specific. They are found consistently in most patients with Hashimoto's thyroiditis but also in a significant number of people with hyper or hypothyroidism.

TSH-R (block) antibodies are often found in thyroiditis without goiter, atrophic thyroiditis accompanied by hypothyroidism. Hashimoto's thyroiditis also has an immune response released by T lymphocytes. Antigen-antibody complexes were observed in the thyroid follicular basal membrane in patients with Hashimoto's thyroiditis. In Hashimoto's thyroiditis there is also a higher incidence than expected of other autoimmune conditions, such as atrophic gastritis and malignant anemia. Also more common is Addison's idiopathic disease, insulin-like diabetes, idiopathic hypoparathyroidism, polyadenal endocrine failure and vitiligo. Hashimoto's thyroiditis often occurs in more people in the same family. Thyroid antibodies are found in 50% of the first-degree relatives of patients with Hashimoto's thyroiditis. The same, however, is observed in relatives of hyperthyroid patients. This indicates that there is a genetically determined predisposition for the disease likely to be associated with the HLA system.

b.ii. Pathological physiology

Thyroid damage is generalized and consists of diffuse and dense lymphocytic infiltration, plasma cell infiltration, rupture of the follicle wall and fibrous tissue growth. The functioning of the gland shows disturbances. The retention of iodine is usually normal, but in some patients it is low, indicative of hypo-function and less high when hyperthyroidism coexists. In these cases, high iodine uptake is not inhibited by thyroid hormones. The binding of iodine to tyrosine is reduced in a large number of patients. The potassium perchlorate delivery test causes an iodine not to be organised and reveals the tyrosine iodination disorders. Because of this disorder and the small thyroid iodine reservoir, the radioiodine retention at 24 hours is often lower than the retention of the first hours. Patients with Hashimoto's thyroiditis are susceptible to the occurrence of hypothyroidism after administration of large doses of iodine, possibly due to the iodine degradation anomaly. Release into the circulation of iodoproteins by thyroid is also common. Thyroid hormones are usually normal or are in the lower normal range until the condition goes into hypothyroidism. Low values exist when gland destruction is important. The level of TSH is often and remains for a long time in the levels of subclinical hypothyroidism.

b.iii. Symptomology

The main symptom of Hashimoto's thyroiditis is swelling of the thyroid. The goiter is installed slowly, is moderate, has uneven surface, it is a lump and semi-consistency. The gland is usually homogeneously inflated due to the superiority of pathological anatomical processes in a certain area. The gland is seldom painful or sensitive to pressure. Pressure phenomena are rare. General phenomena do not exist in Hashimoto's thyroiditis.

b.iv. Laboratory findings

The most typical finding of Hashimoto's thyroiditis is high titers of anti-thyroid antibodies. Anti-TPO antibodies are present in 95% of patients and 60-80% anti-thyroglobulin antibodies. The presence of these antibodies is not pathognomonic for Hashimoto's thyroiditis because the same antibodies are found in a significant number of patients with hyper or hypothyroidism. High titers of antibodies are indicative of thyroiditis. Measuring blood thyroid hormones has no diagnostic value but informs us of hypothyroidism. TSH is usually slightly elevated and is also a good indicator of subclinical hypothyroidism. The radioiodine retention values depend on the functional status of the gland and are not diagnostic. The scintigraphy exhibits heterogeneous retention that reflects the pathological and functional lesions of the parenchyma. Ultrasound is typical in most cases of the disease. It shows an implied inhomogeneity and lobed outline of the gland.

b.v. Diagnosis

The diagnosis of the disease presents problems. In the early stages, the disease is asymptomatic and the swelling of the gland is small. In advanced stages the swelling is noticeable, the surface of the thyroid abnormal and may coexist and symptoms of hypothyroidism. The diagnosis in each phase will mainly be based on the presence of high titer anti-thyroid antibodies. It will be aided by the semi-rigid and nodular or lump of the gland and its ultrasound image. When the title of antibodies is moderately elevated or low, only histological examination may reveal a condition. The hypothyroid status is easily detected by low thyroid hormones and high TSH.

b.vi. Treatment

Treatment of thyroiditis is symptomatic and involves the administration of thyroxine in substitution doses over a long period of time. This treatment is not sure to inhibit the progression of the disease, but it reduces or prevents regressive hyperplasia and covers the body from existing or future hypothyroidism.

c. Riedel's invasive thyroiditis or thyroiditis

Extremely rare form characterized by the development of dense connective tissue, which imparts rocky composition to the gland and filter around the tissues. The etiology of this disease remains unknown. The thyroid is usually swollen and symmetrically filtered by dense fibrous tissue, which destroys the parenchyma. In one third of cases thyroiditis is localized in one lobe. Fiber infiltration extends beyond the thyroid capsule to adjacent tissues, esophagus, trachea and muscles. These infiltrates cause pressures. The onset of the disease is usually gradual. Patients complain about thyroid swelling and stiffness or for compulsive phenomena such as voice gurgling, dysphagia, dyspnoea. Hypothyroidism is rare and is observed when gland destruction is great. The clinical examination reveals a high degree of hardness of the gland. No specific points or laboratory findings exist. The condition resembles thyroid cancer and the diagnosis becomes histological. The treatment is surgery.

8.5 Benign nodules of Thyroid

Benign conditions that can cause thyroid nodule formation include chronic thyroiditis focal areas, a predominant part of a polycystic goiter, cysts from thyroid or parathyroid tissue, or thyroid lining and agenesis of a lobe of the gland with hypertrophy another, which is seen as a cervical mass. Usually the left lobe does not develop and the right one is overturned. The glandular fibrosis after surgery - or the increase of the gland again after surgery or treatment with radioactive iodine - can give a nodular texture. Finally, benign thyroid neoplasms include dilated adenomas, such as colloidal or macrophyllagenic adenomas, embryonic adenomas, embryonic adenomas and Hurthle cell adenomas or acidophils. Rare types of benign lesions include teratomas, lipomas and hemangiomas. Apart from hypertrophy of the right thyroid gland lobe when there is aggression of the left lobe - and some dilated adenomas - all the above lesions are presented as "cold" oozes in isotopic imaging.

The risk factors that predispose to benign or malignant damage are:

• history: a family history of the goiter suggesting benign disease, as well as staying in a region of endemic goiter. Conversely, a family history of myeloid carcinoma, a history of recent thyroid gland enlargement, a voice gullet, dysphagia, or obstruction is a strong indication of cancer.

• Physical characteristics: physical characteristics associated with reduced risk of developing thyroid cancer include older age, female sex, thyroid soft tissues and presence of polycystic goiter. People with a higher risk for thyroid cancer include children, young adults and men. A single hard or dominant nodule, which differs from the rest of the thyroid gland, indicates an increased risk of malignancy. Paralysis of vocal cords, swollen lymph nodes and possible metastases are strong signs of malignancy.

• Serum agents: High titles of serum anti-thyroid antibodies indicate chronic thyroiditis as a cause of thyroid swelling but do not rule out a concomitant malignancy. High serum calcitonin, particularly in patients with a history of myeloid carcinoma, strongly suggests the presence of thyroid cancer. High serum thyroglobulin, after total thyroidectomy for papillary or follicular thyroid cancer, usually indicates metastatic disease, but serum thyroglobulin is not useful in determining the nature of a thyroid hormone.

• imaging methods: Scintigraphic methods can be used to identify "hot" or "cold" oozes, that is, they take up more or less radioactive iodine relative to the surrounding tissue. Hot ouzes are almost never malignant, while colds can be. Thyroid ultrasound can distinguish cystic from solid lesions. A cyst very rarely is malignant. Cystic lesions with internal diaphragms or solid elements may be benign or malignant. CT or MRI may be useful in determining the retrospective extension or localization of thyroid nodes located deep in the cervix.

• needle biopsy: The main development in the treatment of thyroid gland ovary in recent years is the needle biopsy. This technique distinguishes the nodules in three categories: 1. malignant thyroid oesis (95% of thyroid malignancies); 2. breast tumors; 15% of these lesions are malignant and 85% benign, but no cytological distinction can be made; a "warm" mammary neoplasm is benign while a "cold" may be benign or malignant.); 3. benign thyroid oesophageal cancer (exact in 90% of cases - it is seen from surgical procedures or from long- monitoring of patients).

• suppression treatment: benign lesions can be underestimated and sometimes dependent on TSH to a significant extent to shrink to thyroxine treatment. Malignant lesions are unlikely to undermine.

A patient with a thyroid osteoarthritis should be subjected to a needle biopsy. If the brain is malignant, the patient must be referred to the surgery. If the cytology shows that the ovum is benign, the patient is given thyroxine and if the injury subsists then the patient remains on thyroxine indefinitely with a sufficient dose to suppress serum TSH. If there is no regression, a biopsy is performed again. If it increases or changes its composition, it can be removed. Patients in whom the presence of follicular neoplasm has been reported are exposed to radionuclides. If the imaging reveals that the brain is "warm", the patient is simply monitored with or without thyroxine therapy. If the ozone is "cold" and there is an increased likelihood of malignancy, the patient is given thyroxine. If thyroxine does not cause a regurgitation, then the ozone is more likely to be removed.

8.6 Thyroid Cancer

Thyroid cancer stems from thyroid cells that have a wide range of neoplastic transformation. Each histological type of thyroid cancer, papillary carcinoma, follicular, immature and myelogenous has particular features in frequency, progression, prognosis and general biological behavior.

a. Rationale

Thyroid cancer is associated with gene mutations involving genes that are responsible for cell growth and differentiation. The carcinogenicity process is the combination of inactivation of genes that inhibit neoplastic tissue production and activation of oncogenic genes that act on normal or possibly genetically susceptible thyroid cells. In particular, a significant percentage of papillary carcinomas have been found to activate the first-oncogene RET, which causes overexpression of tyrosine kinase leading to neoplastic hyperplasia. In follicular carcinomas, a high incidence of the ras proto-oncogene has been reported which causes permanent stimulation of intracellular substances that contribute to cell growth. Also in follicular carcinomas there is loss of allelic genes of chromosome 3P, which inhibit tumor growth. Undifferentiated anaplastic carcinomas were found to have more frequent mutations of the p53 gene inhibiting tumor growth. Some factors favoring the development of thyroid cancer:

1. The neck irradiation and thyroid exposure to the effects of ionizing radiation causes an increase in thyroid cancer incidence.

2. Prolonged TSH administration or increased endogenous TSH following administration of bronchoconstrictors or iodine-poor food causes thyroid cancer in experimental animals. However, the transfer of these observations to humans is difficult.

3. Thyroid myeloid carcinoma is familial in nature and this prejudices the existence of hereditary predisposition for this type of cancer.

b. Symptomology

The main symptom of thyroid cancer is swelling of the gland. Following are the infiltration of the cervical glands, the symptoms of pressure and complications from metastases. The swelling may be small and circumscribed and be in the form of a lump which, for a number of years, remains unchanged in volume or texture or increases slowly. In other cases the swelling is large with a rapid increase, which quickly occupies the whole gland as it does in tumors. The surface of the swelling is usually abnormal and swollen and the texture is harsh and sometimes stony. However, palpation of either swollen or soft swelling does not exclude the existence of cancer because the healthy tissue surrounding the neoplasm changes the palpable characters of the tumor. The presence of palpable lateral cervical lymph nodes combined with swelling of the gland leads to the conclusion of thyroid carcinoma. Pressure symptoms are characteristic of carcinoma and rarely occur in other situations. Consisting in swallowing, hoarseness of the voice, the difficulty in breathing. Metastasis sometimes gives symptoms first. Persistent diarrhea, lasting months or years, is seen in myeloid thyroid carcinoma sufferers.

c. Laboratory findings

Thyroid cancer patients maintain normal functioning of the healthy part of the gland. For this reason, thyroid function control gives normal values. The diagnosis of the neoplasm contributes to the scintigraphy, ultrasound, radiological control and, in particular, the puncture and biopsy of the filtered lymph nodes. Thyroid scintigraphy reveals, respectively, the palpable swelling of a deficient image or reduced retention of the radioisotope due to its ingestion from the neoplastic tissue. The cold area is a part of the lobe or the entire lobe and has a characteristic abnormal edge. In some cases, the neoplasm is small or covered by a thick layer of normal thyroid parenchyma so that its presence in the scintigraphy is not recognized because of the radiation of the tissue that covers it. The scintigraphy also serves to detect metastases when they are large enough and have adequate intake to be depicted in the scintigraphy. The ultrasound provides information on the extent and especially morphology and swelling and has the advantage that it can be repeated infinitely without consequences for the patient and thus helps to monitor the development of a swelling. Control by modern imaging methods allows us to detect anomalies due to pressure that may be due to thyroid tumor growth. It also contributes to the detection of bone metastases, which are perceived by osteolytic processes that cause both pulmonary metastases, which have a characteristic image. Puncture of a needle with a fine needle has a diagnostic value only on a positive result when atypical cells are found. The puncture of the filtered cervical glands and the detection of carcinoma cells often puts the diagnosis of the primary outbreak, located in the thyroid. Measurable blood calcitonin, which is very much increased in myeloid carcinoma and anti-thyroid antibodies, which, when found in high titers, advocate Hashimoto's thyroiditis.

d. Diagnosis

Clinical-laboratory investigation of a thyroid swelling rarely carries a diagnosis of cancer safely. An exception is the positive effect of fine needle puncture and the finding of metastases that receive the radioiodine. In other cases the test results simply make more or less likely the presence of a malignant neoplasm. Thyroid cancer is diagnosed with a histological examination, which in addition to the detection of malignancy will also determine the type of carcinoma, which is important because once we know the type of cancer, the treatment depends on the highly biological characteristics of the various forms of carcinoma. The prognosis of thyroid cancer is not as unfavorable as in other cancers. It depends on the type of cancer and on the evolutionary stage.

Chapter 9: Thyroid diet plan

The hormones secreted from the thyroid gland are thyroxine (T4) and tryiodothyronine (T3). T3 is the active hormone and T4 acts as the prohormone. Only 20% of T3 is secreted from the thyroid and rest 80% comes from T4 deiodination in peripheral organs like liver and kidney. Thyroid hormone regulates metabolic rate, body temperature and tissue growth.

The thyroid hormone synthesis :
- active uptake of circulating iodide to cytosol by sodium iodide symporter
- oxidation of iodide by thyroid peroxidase and iodination of tyrosine residues on thyroglobulin molecule, creating mono and diiodotyrosines
- coupling of iodinated tyrosine residues to form T3 and T4
- proteolysis due to hydrolysis and releasing the T3 and T4 in cytosol.

As it is obvious Iodine is the major nutrient required for the synthesis of thyroid hormones. As the second most important nutrient remains the selenium, which forms selenocysteine compounds and protects the thyroid from free radical damage. Furthermore, as important in hormone synthesis are iron, vitamin A and zinc Hence, dietary intake of all these nutrients is essential for the correct functioning of the thyroid gland.

Iodine is important for the iodination of tyrosine residues leading to the formation of thyroid hormones. Environmental iodine is the main source of iodine, that is present in soil, sea water, dairy products, seafood and eggs. Recommended dietary allowance for iodine for adults is 150 ug and for pregnant and lactating women is 220 ug and 290 ug respectively. Urinary iodine level is the best measure to assess the iodine level in the body. Deficiency of iodine is diagnosed when the median concentration is less than 50 ug/ml.

Selenium is a critical enzyme in thyroid hormone synthesis. Selenoproteins are responsible for the cellular antioxidative defense and protects the thyroid gland from damage due to hydrogen peroxide and reactive oxygen species. Also, selenoproteins are involved in the activation and inactivation of thyroid hormones. Selenium is found mainly in the soil and selenium rich foods are mushrooms, garlic, onions, eggs, beef liver, shellfish, wheat germ, sunflower seeds and sesame seeds.

Iron is essential for normal thyroid hormone metabolism.

Below we summarize all the food important in a healthy diet for the correct function of thyroid gland and some food to avoid.

Consider eating more...

- Seaweed

If your thyroid needs more iodine in order to work properly and produce enough TH for your body's needs. Many types of seaweed are chockfull of iodine, but the amount can vary wildly.

- Yogurt

Dairy products are full of this. Part of the reason is because livestock are given iodine supplements and the milking process involves iodine-based cleaners. Plain, low-fat yogurt, or Greek yogurt is a good source—it can make up about 50% of your daily intake of iodine.

- Brazil nuts

Brazil nuts are packed with another nutrient that helps regulate thyroid hormones: selenium. It is recommended in order to get the daily dose of selenium, a trace mineral that's highly concentrated in the thyroid gland and plays an essential role in thyroid hormone production. Also, it may also help stave off long-term thyroid damage in people with thyroid-related problems like Hashimoto's and Graves' disease.

- Milk

Much of the iodine comes from dairy products. By drinking 1 cup of low-fat milk, you'll consume about one-third of your daily iodine needs. People with hypothyroidism were more likely to be deficient in D than their healthier counterparts.

- Chicken and beef

Zinc is another key nutrient for your thyroid—your body needs it to churn out TH. Take in too little zinc, and it can lead to hypothyroidism. But get this: If you develop hypothyroidism, you can also become deficient in zinc, since your thyroid hormones help absorb the mineral.

- Fish

Since iodine is found in soils and seawater, fish is a good source.

- Shellfish

Shellfish like lobster and shrimp are good sources of iodine. In fact, just 3 ounces of shrimp (about 4 or 5 pieces) contains more than 20% of your recommended intake.

- Eggs

One large egg contains about 16% of the iodine and 20% of the selenium you need for the day, making them a thyroid superfood.

- Salmon

Some findings suggest that many people with Hashimoto's disease (the most common type of hypothyroidism) have lower levels of vitamin D That's bad news, since low D is tied to higher levels of thyroid antibodies.

Getting the recommended 600 IUs of vitamin D per day can keep some of that inflammation at bay so your thyroid can function at its best. And salmon is a top source, with 570 IUs per 3-ounce serving

- White beans

A cup of cooked white beans serves up 8mg of iron—a mineral that many people, especially premenopausal women, have trouble getting enough. First, iron is tough for the body to absorb, but you can boost your absorption of iron-rich foods by pairing them with a source of vitamin C. And second, iron can make thyroid drugs less efficient. So be sure to take your thyroid meds at least four hours before or after eating an iron-rich meal.

Consider eating less...

- Soy

Eating the wrong soy foods—or having too much soy in general—can spell bad news for your thyroid. The mineral iodine is an essential building block for thyroid hormone, but soy contains isoflavone compounds that block iodine from doing its job.

Most people with hypothyroidism don't need to steer clear of soy completely. But it's a good idea to limit your consumption to a few servings a week, and to stick with minimally processed forms of soy like tempeh or miso. Foods containing processed soy protein isolates tend to have a higher concentration of isoflavones.

- Cruciferous veggies

Broccoli, cauliflower, Brussels sprouts, and cabbage. Even though they're loaded with nutrition, cruciferous vegetables are also high in naturally occurring enzymes called goitrogens, which can interfere with the production of thyroid hormone.

- Gluten

Gluten-containing foods like wheat, barley, and rye can trigger inflammation.

- Processed foods

More than 75% of our dietary sodium intake comes from restaurant, pre-packaged, and processed fare. But manufacturers don't have to use iodized salt in their products. You may be taking in too much sodium (which can set you up for high blood pressure, then heart disease), minus the iodine.

- Fast food

Fast food chains also aren't required to use iodized salt in their foods. And even when they do, it might not boost the iodine content all that much.

CONCLUSION

Thank you for purchasing this book. The idea of writing it, came from a friend of mine who suffers from thyroid problems. That is the reason I took the decision to search as much as I could to help him. After many hours of studying, I realized that my level of knowledge as far as the thyroid gland is concerned is very high, so I tried to write my very first book! I managed to do it and here we are. Special thanks to Sofia Vatsiou who helped me to write the book.

www.ingramcontent.com/pod-product-compliance
Lightning Source LLC
Chambersburg PA
CBHW021829170526
45157CB00007B/2729